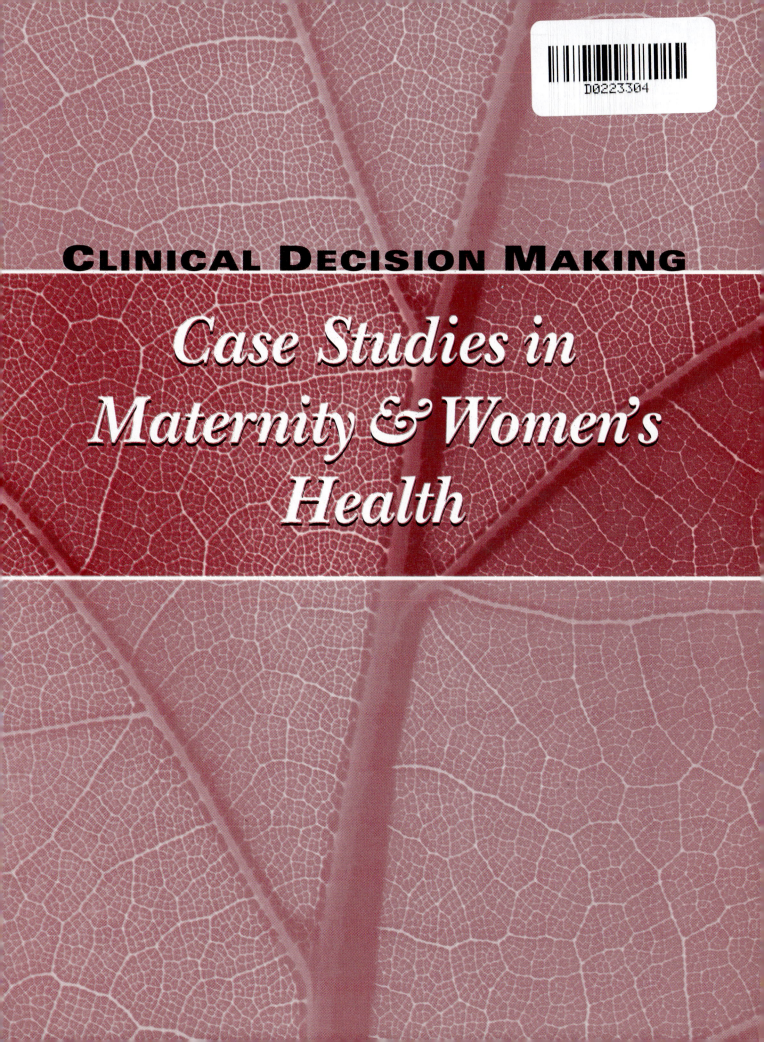

CLINICAL DECISION MAKING

Case Studies in Maternity & Women's Health

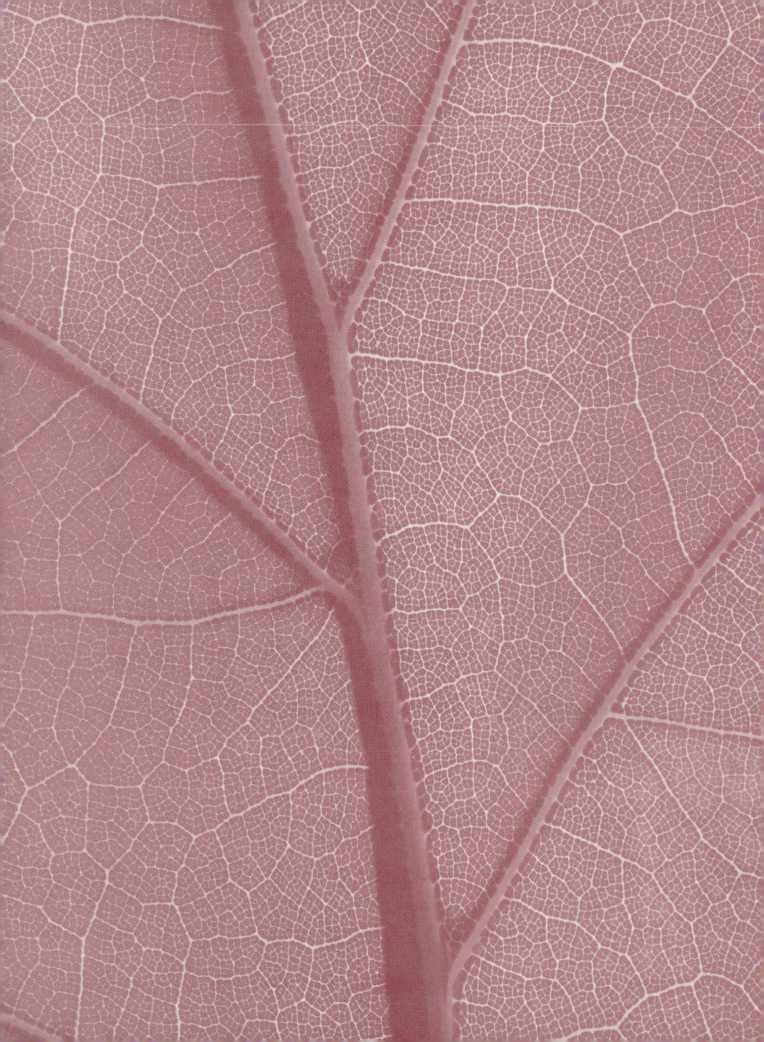

CLINICAL DECISION MAKING

Case Studies in Maternity & Women's Health

Diann S. Gregory
ARNP, CNM, MSEd

Professor of Nursing
MIAMI DADE COLLEGE, MIAMI, FLORIDA

THOMSON

DELMAR LEARNING™

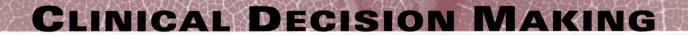

Australia   Canada   Mexico   Singapore   Spain   United Kingdom   United States

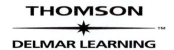

Clinical Decision Making: Case Studies in Maternity and Women's Health
by Diann S. Gregory

Vice President, Health Care Business Unit:
William Brottmiller

Editorial Director:
Cathy L. Esperti

Executive Editor:
Matthew Kane

Developmental Editor:
Maria D'Angelico

Editorial Assistant:
Michelle Leavitt

Marketing Director:
Jennifer McAvey

Production Director:
Carolyn Miller

Production Editor:
Jack Pendleton

Library of Congress Cataloging-in-Publication Data

Gregory, Diann S.
   Clinical decision making : case studies in maternity and women's health / Diann S. Gregory.
      p. ; cm.
   Includes bibliographical references and index.
   ISBN 1-4018-2709-8 (pbk.)
   1. Maternity nursing—Decision making—Case studies. 2. Gynecologic nursing—Decision making—Case studies. 3. Maternity nursing—Problems, exercises, etc. 4. Gynecologic nursing—Problems, exercises, etc.
   [DNLM: 1. Maternal-Child Nursing—methods—Case Reports. 2. Maternal-Child Nursing—methods—Problems and Exercises. 3. Cultural Diversity—Case Reports. 4. Cultural Diversity—Problems and Exercises. 5. Nursing Assessment—Case Reports. 6. Nursing Assessment—Problems and Exercises. 7. Women's Health—Case Reports. 8. Women's Health—Problems and Exercises.—WY 18.2 G822c 2006]
   I. Title.
   RG951.G74 2006
   618.1'0231—dc22

                                          2005005297

Notice to the Reader

Contents

Reviewers

Denise G. Link, NPC, DNSc
Women's Health Care Nurse Practitioner
Clinical Associate Professor
Arizona State University
Tempe, Arizona

Tamella Livengood, APRN, BC, MSN, FNP
Nursing Faculty, Northwestern Michigan College
Traverse City, Michigan

Vicki Nees, RNC, MSN, APRN-BC
Associate Professor
Ivy Tech State College
Lafayette, Indiana

Patricia Posey-Goodwin, MSN, RN, EdD (c)
Assistant Professor
University of West Florida
Pensacola, Florida

Series Preface

Thomson Delmar Learning's Case Studies Series was created to encourage nurses to bridge the gap between content knowledge and clinical application. The products within the series represent the most innovative and comprehensive approach to nursing case studies ever developed. Each title has been authored by experienced nurse educators and clinicians who understand the complexity of nursing practice as well as the challenges of teaching and learning. All of the cases are based on real-life clinical scenarios and demand thought and "action" from the nurse. Each case brings the user into the clinical setting and invites the reader to utilize the nursing process while considering all of the variables that influence the client's condition and the care to be provided. Each case also represents a unique set of variables to offer a breadth of learning experiences and to capture the reality of nursing practice. To gauge the progression of a user's knowledge and critical thinking ability, the cases have been categorized by difficulty level. Every section begins with basic cases and proceeds to more advanced scenarios, thereby presenting opportunities for learning and practice for both students and professionals.

All of the cases have been reviewed by experts to ensure that as many variables as possible are represented in a truly realistic manner and that each case reflects consistency with realities of modern nursing practice.

How to Use This Book

Every case begins with a table of variables that are encountered in practice and that must be understood by the nurse in order to provide appropriate care to the client. Categories of variables include age, setting, ethnicity, cultural considerations, pre-existing conditions, co-existing conditions, communication considerations, disability considerations, socioeconomic considerations, spiritual considerations, pharmacological considerations, psychosocial considerations, legal considerations, ethical considerations, alternative therapy, prioritization considerations, and delegation considerations. If a case involves a variable that is considered to have a significant impact on care, the specific variable is included in the table. This allows the user an "at a glance" view of the issues that will need to be considered to provide care to the client in the scenario. The table of variables is followed by a presentation of the case, including the history of the client, current condition, clinical setting, and professionals involved. A series of questions follows each case that ask the users to consider how they would handle the issues presented within the scenario. Suggested answers and rationales are provided for remediation and discussion.

Organization

The cases are grouped into parts based on topics. Within each part, cases are organized by difficulty level from easy, to moderate, to difficult. The classifications are somewhat subjective, but they are based upon a developed standard. In general, difficulty level has been determined by the number of variables that impact the case and the complexity of the client's condition. Colored tabs are used to allow the user to distinguish the difficulty levels more easily. A comprehensive table of variables is also provided for reference to allow the user to quickly select cases containing a particular variable of care.

Praise for Thomson Delmar Learning's Case Study Series

I would recommend this book to my undergraduate students. This would be a required book for graduate students in nursing education, women's health, or maternal–child programs.

PATRICIA POSEY-GOODWIN, MSN, RN, EdD (C)
Assistant Professor
University of West Florida

This text does an excellent job of reflecting the complexity of nursing practice.

VICKI NEES, RNC, MSN, APRN-BC
Associate Professor
Ivy Tech State College

. . . [T]he case studies are very comprehensive and allow the undergraduate student an opportunity to apply knowledge gained in the classroom to a potentially real clinical situation.

TAMELLA LIVENGOOD, APRN, BC, MSN, FNP
Nursing Faculty
Northwestern Michigan College

I commend the effort to include the impact of illness on the growth and development of the child, on the family's cohesiveness, and on the subsequent health problems that will affect the child in years to come. Inclusion of questions that focus on the nurse's perceptions, biases, and beliefs are extremely important when training nurses to provide comprehensive care . . . Often one system illness will affect another health system, and this has been demonstrated numerous times [in this text].

DIANA JACOBSON
MS, RN, CPNP
Faculty Associate
Arizona State University College of Nursing

These cases and how you have approached them definitely stimulate the students to use critical-thinking skills. I thought the questions asked really pushed the students to think deeply and thoroughly.

JOANNE SOLCHANY, PhD, ARNP, RN, CS
Assistant Professor, Family & Child Nursing
University of Washington

The use of case studies is pedagogically sound and very appealing to students and instructors. I think that some instructors avoid them because of the challenge of case development. You have provided the material for them.

NANCY L. OLDENBURG, RN, MS, CPNP
Clinical Instructor
Northern Illinois University

[The author] has done an excellent job of assisting students to engage in critical thinking. I am very impressed with the cases, questions, and content. I rarely ask that students buy more than one pediatrics book . . . but, in this instance, I can't wait until this book is published.

DEBORAH J. PERSELL, MSN, RN, CPNP
Assistant Professor
Arkansas State University

This is a groundbreaking book that . . . will be appropriate for undergraduate pediatric courses as well as a variety of graduate programs. . . . One of the most impressive features is the variety of cases that cover situations from primary care through critical care and rehabilitation. The cases are presented to develop and assess critical-thinking skills. . . . All cases are framed within a comprehensive presentation of physical findings, stimulating critical thinking about pathophysiology, developmental considerations, and family systems. This book should be a required text for all undergraduate and graduate nursing programs and should be well-received by faculty.

JANE H. BARNSTEINER, PhD, RN, FAAN
Professor of Pediatric Nursing
University of Pennsylvania School of Nursing

Preface

Clinical Decision Making: Case Studies in Maternity and Women's Health has been developed to provide the student with an opportunity to experience a wide range of clinical encounters in women's health. The case format provides the opportunity to move from theory to application. It provides instructors with a transitional tool to guide students into practice. Currently, many programs have reduced the time devoted to specialty areas. This makes it nearly impossible for clinical instructors to provide the many learning experiences needed by the student. The case studies format gives students the opportunity to utilize the nursing process in order to make decisions based on multiple variables. The clients, although fictitious, are presented as believable characters in multicultural, realistic scenarios, removing as much as possible the situations from isolated text theory and asking students to relate to the persons as individuals. It is the intention that adding this realism will guide the student into focusing on the whole person and her responses to health changes, not merely on the physical processes.

Empowerment of women and their families is maintained as an essential core in this process. Currently, providers of maternity care are faced with the high risk associated with malpractice suits and financial constraints as a result of reduced reimbursement and increased insurance cost. This often results in pressure to provide "medical-legal" care. The nurse, practicing the advocacy role, provides the balance that keeps care client-centered. Often this is difficult because nursing itself struggles with downsizing and short staffing. A concerted effort has been made to apply current evidence-based science and to guide readers into the exploration of both short-term and long-term effects of routine non-evidence-based interventions. Nurses who have a confident grasp of evidence-based care are better prepared to intervene for their client's well-being. Readers are encouraged to stay current on newer evidence-based studies as they are released and revisit cases to apply this knowledge as it becomes available.

Organization

Cases are grouped according to phases in the childbearing cycle. Prenatal cases are presented initially, followed by intrapartum, newborn, and then postpartum. These are followed by cases in non-maternity-related women's health. The cases are fictitious; however, they are based on actual problems and/or situations the nurse will encounter throughout a career in Women's Health. Any resemblance to actual cases or individuals is coincidental.

To assist the instructor in assigning cases, each case is preceded by a blueprint listing the specific variables being presented in the case. For example, the following information is listed when it is pertinent for that case: Client age, setting, ethnicity, significant history factors, pre-existing conditions, co-existing conditions, communication problems, disabilities, socioeconomic factors, spiritual or religious factors, prioritization concerns, legal and ethical concerns, need for delegation, pharmacologic agents, and alternative therapies referred to in the case. The level of difficulty is identified at the start of the case, and a brief overview is provided.

The case is then presented, starting with a client profile to provide background, followed by the scenario. Each scenario is followed by a series of questions. The instructor's manual that accompanies the text contains the answers, rationales, and references.

In addition to cases that focus on the client disease and responses to disease, the scenarios are presented in multicultural settings, which present real ethical and moral dilemmas that nurses are facing in the workplace and the community. In the more advanced cases the student is asked to utilize critical thinking, apply the nursing process, and use professional judgment to critique the care provided. Students are asked to review routine interventions in light of evidence-based studies for both evidence efficacy and the impact of these interventions on safety and the quality of the care provided.

Several cases present social problems reflecting flaws in the current provider networks. The student is presented with clients who have "fallen through the cracks" in the system and is asked to explore ways that the professional nurse can become proactive to bring about social change for better delivery of care.

Acknowledgments

My sincere thanks to Maria D'Angelico, Developmental Editor, and the entire editorial staff at Thomson Delmar Learning for guidance in writing this text and making it a reality. A special thank you to Justine Clegg for reviewing the case on grieving. Justine's years of experience as both a certified professional midwife and mental health counselor were valuable to completing this case. Thank you to Heather Gordon for reviewing and contributing to several of the well woman and neonatal cases. I would also like to thank the reviewers for their time and valuable input.

Dedication

This book is dedicated to my husband, John, our children, and their families for their continued support and encouragement through this very long process. A special dedication of this book goes to Janice Heller, CPM and my friend, and to the many dedicated midwives and nurses who still believe in normal birth and who have spent a lifetime empowering women who seek holistic family-centered care and out-of-hospital birth. As long as you are out there, normal birth will be safe.

About the Author

Diann S. Gregory received her BSN at Madonna University in 1969. Diann's grandmother Robertson guided her in the direction of nursing and her mother's courage and dad's challenge made it possible to go to college. She received her MSEd in adult education from Florida International University, and her Nurse Midwifery Certificate in 1998 from the Frontier School of Nursing and Midwifery (CNEP program).

Diann started her nursing career in the Army Nurse Corps as an operating room nurse in Viet Nam, where she received a bronze star for her work in surgery and volunteer work at the local orphanage.

She has spent over 36 years working as a staff nurse, patient educator, clinical specialist, and nursing faculty at the associate and bachelor's level and has been a preceptor at the masters level in the field of Women's Health. For the past 12 years she has taught direct entry midwifery at Miami Dade College. Diann earned her RNC in 1986 from the NAACOG Certification Corp. and is a Lamaze certified instructor. Over the past nine years on three different occasions, Diann has been honored by her peers to receive the highest honor awarded to Miami Dade College professors, the three-year Endowed Teaching Chair. She has also twice been awarded the NISOD award for teaching excellence from the University of Texas at Austin. Recently she was recognized as a finalist in The Thomas Ehrlich Faculty Award for Service-Learning, an annual national award that recognizes leaders in community service learning.

Her contributions to education include authoring several video teaching tapes in the series "ABC of Nursing" produced at Miami Dade College, one of which, "Intrapartum Care," received first place from the National League for Nursing in 1993. Through grants she created and developed interactive virtual practices for teaching antepartum to midwifery students. This program has been presented at several national conferences. She was instrumental in obtaining grants to develop a program to train doulas and has her own consulting business working with hospitals in the areas of quality assurance and risk management. For over 20 years Diann has worked as a legal consultant to legal firms in three counties. She is currently a full-time professor in the nursing and midwifery programs at Miami Dade College.

Diann married her combat buddy from Viet Nam. John was a medical evacuation DUSTOFF helicopter pilot, and is her lifetime hero. They dated in combat boots and he won her heart as he would daily put the lives of the soldiers in the field above his own as he headed into active combat zones to bring them into her hospital. They have been married for 34 years and have four children.

Diann has been blessed to be doula for their daughter Diann and husband, Dan, during their three difficult high-risk deliveries. On the request of her daughter-in-law, two years ago she flew to Korea where their son John, an Army officer, was stationed. There she was honored to be the midwife to her daughter-in-law, Yali, and guided her through the birth of a granddaughter. John and Yali's five-year-old daughter provided assistance. John and Diann's youngest daughter, Josie, and husband, Sam, look forward to her support in the near future as they plan their family. John and Diann's youngest, Tony, has proudly become a Florida Gator this year as he enters his junior year at the University of Florida in the electrical engineering program. Family has filled Diann's life with love that she has been able to bring to each of her clients and students over many years.

Diann may be reached at Miami Dade College, Medical Center Campus, 950 NW 20th Street, Miami, Florida 33127. She may also be contacted by e-mail at dgregory@mdc.edu or by phone at 305 237-4460.

Comprehensive Table
of Variables

CASE STUDY	AGE	SETTING	CULTURAL CONSIDERATIONS	ETHNICITY	PRE-EXISTING CONDITION	CO-EXISTING CONDITION/CURRENT PROBLEM	COMMUNICATIONS	DISABILITY	SOCIOECONOMIC STATUS	SPIRITUAL/RELIGIOUS	PSYCHOSOCIAL	LEGAL	ETHICAL	PRIORITIZATION	DELEGATION	PHARMACOLOGIC	ALTERNATIVE THERAPY	SIGNIFICANT HISTORY
Part 1: Prenatal Case Studies																		
1	23	Midwifery private practice		White American		x					x					x		x
2	17	Indian Reservation Clinic	Native American traditions	Native American					x	x	x					x		x
3	23	Certified Nurse Midwifery office	Recent Nigerian immigrant	African	x	x	x				x			x				x
4	36	Birth center	Rural American culture	White American	x	x							x	x				
5	Adolescent	Prenatal clinic	Rastafarian Jamaican traditions	Jamaican														
6	43	Women's clinic	White middle-class American culture	White American	x	x												x
7	26	Prenatal clinic	Caribbean culture	Hispanic American	x								x	x		x		
8	23	Private prenatal office	Mexican traditional health beliefs	Hispanic American													x	x
9	36	Free clinic		White American	x	x	x		x		x		x			x		x
10	16	Prenatal clinic		White American		x					x	x						
11	28	Birth center prenatal clinic	Native American traditions	Native American	x				x	x								x
Part 2: Intrapartum Case Studies																		
1	19	Certified Nurse Midwifery office/phone triage	Middle-class White American culture	White American	x		x										x	x
2	29	Home		White American		x												x
3	15	Hospital urgent care center	Puerto Rican traditional beliefs	Hispanic American	x	x	x	x				x		x		x		x
4	23	Private OB practice/hospital	Traditional Colombian culture	Colombian	x	x	x						x					x
5	21	Freestanding birth center		White American														x
6	24	Birth center to hospital transfer	Black-Muslim traditions	Black American	x	x	x			x								x
7	36	Hospital labor and delivery unit		Indonesian American	x	x	x									x		x
8	41	Hospital labor and delivery unit		White American		x				x			x			x	x	x

#	Age/Time	Setting	Cultural context	Ethnicity	1	2	3	4	5	6	7	8	9	10	11
9	26	Birth center	American urban professional culture	White American		x		x	x						x
10	17	Hospital labor and delivery unit	Black American	Black American		x		x			x			x	x
11		Hospital labor unit		Varied		x					x		x	x	
12	22	Hospital labor and delivery unit	Accepts American medicalization concepts of pregnancy and birth	Black American		x		x				x			x

Part 3: Newborn Case Studies

#	Age/Time	Setting	Cultural context	Ethnicity	1	2	3	4	5	6	7	8	9	10	11
1	24 hours	Hospital postpartum unit		White American		x								x	x
2	Newborn	Hospital delivery room		Black American		x			x						x
3	18 hours	Postpartum unit	Cuban American immigrant traditions	Cuban		x			x					x	x
4	6 hours	Small community hospital nursery		Black American	x	x									x
5	48 hours	Home		Black American		x			x						x
6	24 hours	Newborn nursery		White American		x								x	x
7	3 hours	Hospital		White American	x	x								x	x
8	2 hours	Hospital NB nursery		White American		x									x

Part 4: Postpartum Case Studies

#	Age/Time	Setting	Cultural context	Ethnicity	1	2	3	4	5	6	7	8	9	10	11
1	29	Hospital postpartum unit	White American culture	White American		x		x							x
2	23	Home		White American		x								x	x
3	24	Home	Cuban traditions	Cuban American		x		x						x	x
4	14	Clinic		White American		x		x							x
5	26	Hospital postpartum unit	Pakistani traditions	Pakistani			x	x							x
6	24	Hospital postpartum unit	Jamaican Rastafarian culture	Black American	x	x			x					x	x

Part 5: Well Woman Case Studies

#	Age/Time	Setting	Cultural context	Ethnicity	1	2	3	4	5	6	7	8	9	10	11
1	15	Certified Nurse Midwife's office		White American	x	x			x	x	x	x			
2	28	Women's clinic		Black American		x									x
3	36	Well Woman clinic		Black American		x								x	x
4	31	Certified Nurse Midwife's office		Hispanic American		x								x	x x
5	36	Infertility specialty center	Shinto health beliefs	Asian American	x	x		x	x	x		x		x	x x
6	48	Well Woman private clinic	Black American professional culture	Black American	x	x		x		x				x	x x
7	68	Well Woman clinic	Advanced age	White American	x	x	x	x	x	x				x	x

Abbreviations Commonly Used in Maternity and Women's Health Nursing

ABR . . . . auditory brainstem response
AFI . . . . amniotic fluid index
AFP . . . . alpha fetoprotein
AGCUS . . . . atypical glandular cells of undetermined significance
AMA . . . . advanced maternal age
AROM . . . . artificial rupture of membranes
ARNP . . . . advance registered nurse practitioner
ASCUS . . . . atypical squamous cells of undetermined significance
BMI . . . . body mass index
BMR . . . . basal metabolic rate
BP . . . . blood pressure
BPD . . . . bronchopulmonary dysplasia
BPP . . . . biophysical profile
BTBV . . . . beat to beat variability
BV . . . . bacterial vaginosis
CBC . . . . complete blood count
CNM . . . . certified nurse midwife
CVAT . . . . costovertebral angle tenderness
CVS . . . . chorionic villus sampling
CPD . . . . cephalopelvic disproportion
CPM . . . . certified professional midwife
DIC . . . . disseminated intravascular coagulopathy
DVT . . . . deep vein thrombosis
EBL . . . . estimated blood loss
EFW . . . . estimated fetal weight
EOAD . . . . evoked otoacoustic emission test
FH . . . . fundal height
FHT . . . . fetal heart tone
FM . . . . fetal movement
fob . . . . father of the baby
FSE . . . . fetal scalp electrode

FSH . . . . follicle-stimulating hormone
FTP . . . . failure to progress
GBS . . . . group B streptococcus
hCG . . . . human chorionic gonadotropin
H&H . . . . hematocrit and hemoglobin
H&P . . . . history and physical
HA . . . . headache
HELLP . . . . hemolysis elevated liver enzymes and low platelets
HRT . . . . hormone replacement therapy
HSIL . . . high-grade squamous intraepithelial lesions
I&O . . . . intake and output
IDM . . . . infant of diabetic mother
IUGR . . . . intrauterine growth retardation
IUP . . . . intrauterine pregnancy
IUPC . . . . intrauterine pressure catheter
KVO . . . . keep vein open
LLQ . . . . left lower quadrant
LNMP . . . . last normal menstrual period
LOA . . . . left occiput anterior
LSB . . . . lower sternal border
LSIL . . . . . low-grade squamous intraepithelial lesions
LTV . . . . long-term variablility
MAS . . . . meconium aspiration syndrome
MMS . . . . multiple marker screening
NEC . . . . necrotizing enterocolitis
NST . . . . non-stress test
NSVD . . . . normal spontaneous vaginal delivery
OCP . . . . oral contraceptive pills
ONTD . . . . open neural tube defects
PDA . . . . patent ductus arteriosis
PID . . . . pelvic inflammatory disease

PMI . . . . point of maximal impulse

PPV. . . . . positive pressure ventilation

PPW . . . . pre-pregnancy weight

PPROM. . . . . preterm premature rupture of membranes

PROM. . . . . premature rupture of membranes

PTL. . . . . preterm labor

RDS. . . . . respiratory distress syndrome

R/O . . . . rule out

r/t . . . . related to

S < D. size less than dates

SIDS . . . . sudden infant death syndrome

SIL . . . . squamous intraepithelial lesions

SROM . . . . spontaneous rupture of membranes

STI. . . . sexually transmitted infection (also known as STD—sexually transmitted disease)

T . . . . temperature

TENS . . . . transcutaneous electrical nerve stimulator

Toc. . . . . test of cure

TOP . . . . termination of pregnancy

TPN. . . . . total parenteral nutrition

TTN . . . . transient tachypnea of the newborn

URQ . . . . upper right quadrant

UTI . . . . urinary tract infection

VBAC. . . . . vaginal birth after cesarean

VE. . . . . vaginal exam

VS. . . . . vital signs

wga . . . . weeks gestational age

wnl . . . . within normal limit

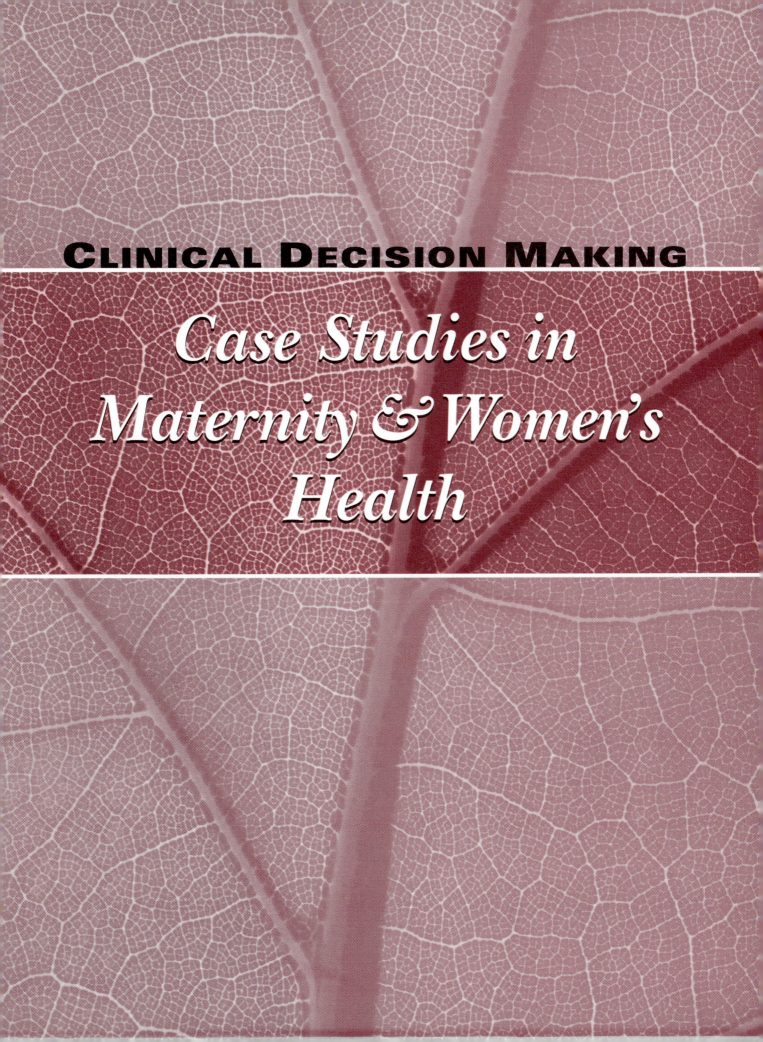

CLINICAL DECISION MAKING

Case Studies in Maternity & Women's Health

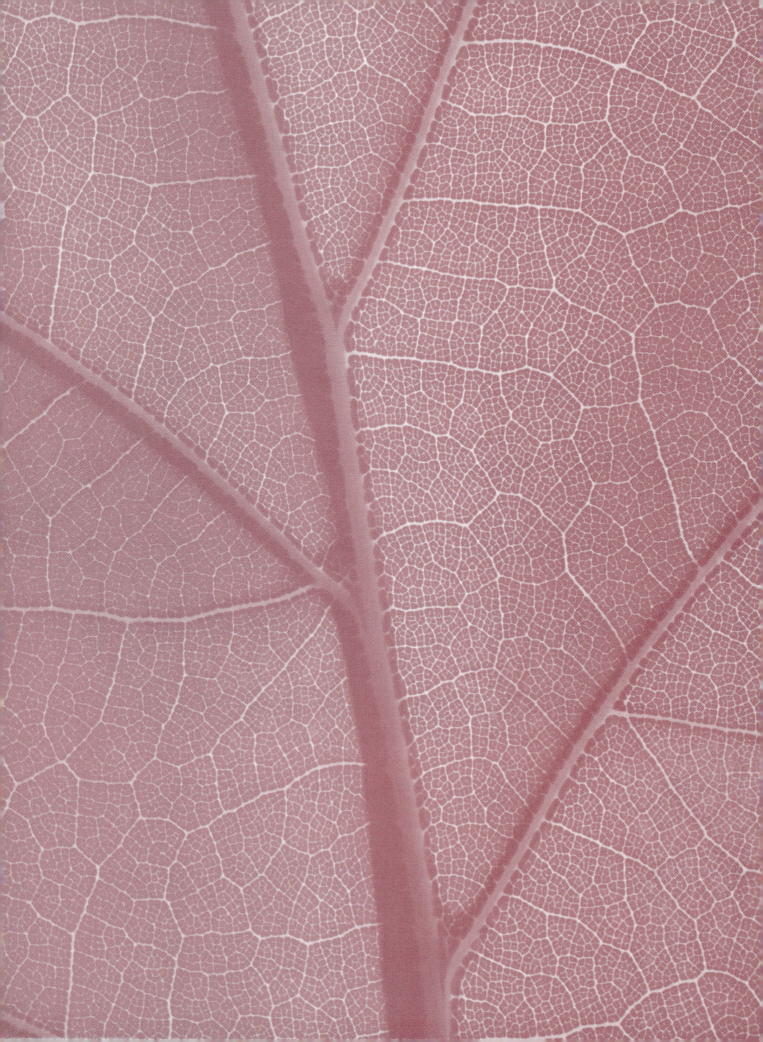

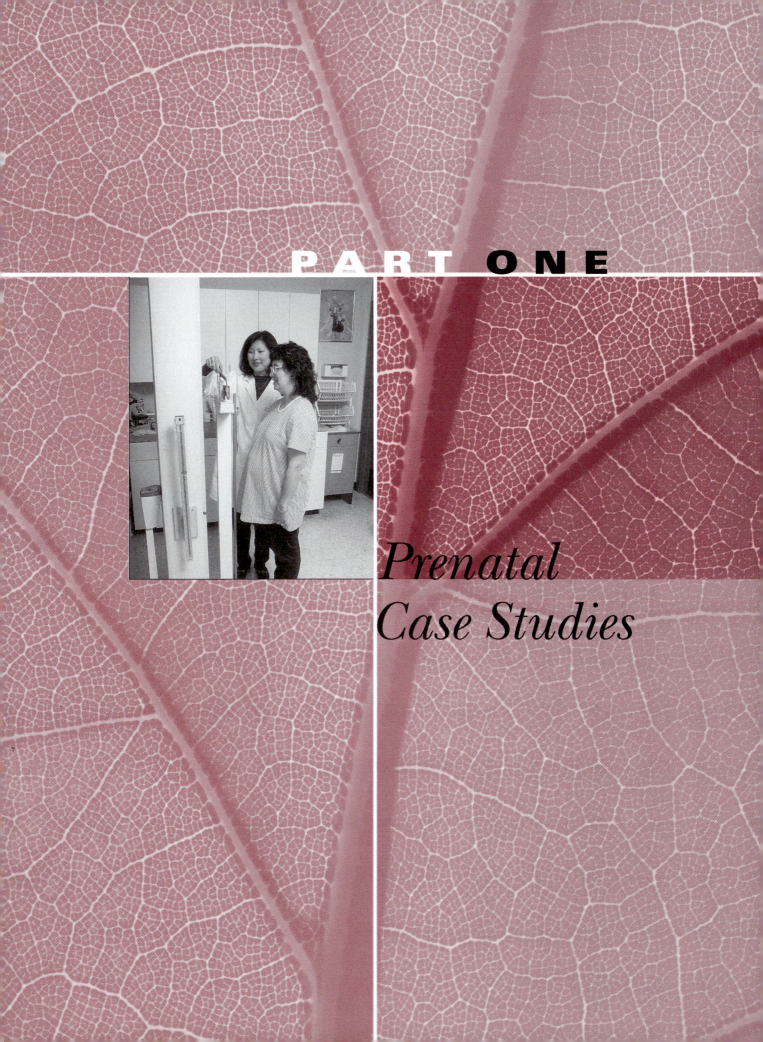

PART ONE

*Prenatal
Case Studies*

Linda

AGE

23

SETTING

- Midwifery private practice

CULTURAL CONSIDERATIONS

ETHNICITY

- White American

PRE-EXISTING CONDITION

CO-EXISTING CONDITION/CURRENT PROBLEM

- Pregnant while taking oral contraceptives

COMMUNICATIONS

DISABILITY

SOCIOECONOMIC STATUS

SPIRITUAL/RELIGIOUS

PSYCHOSOCIAL

- Trauma related to preterm birth/neonatal death

LEGAL

ETHICAL

PRIORITIZATION

DELEGATION

PHARMACOLOGIC

- Metronidazole (Flagyl)
- Oral contraceptives

ALTERNATIVE THERAPY

SIGNIFICANT HISTORY

- Termination of pregnancy; preterm birth/neonatal death; multigravida

PRENATAL, second trimester

Level of difficulty: Easy

Overview: This case asks the student to respond to the mother regarding common changes that occur in pregnancy. It also asks the student to assess any risks associated with the mother using hormonal birth control during the early months of pregnancy.

Client Profile

Linda is a 23-year-old, married, White female (MWF). Linda went to see her family doctor after she had experienced two months of nausea and vomiting. She had been on birth control pills for two years and was certain that she could not be pregnant. The physician did a pregnancy test, and it was positive. Linda had often skipped periods when taking the pill and did not consider three months without a period unusual. She had been pregnant twice before. The first time was when she was 15 years old, and she had a first trimester elective abortion. The second time was three years ago, when she experienced a preterm birth at 28 weeks, and the baby died shortly after birth. That was a very traumatic experience for her, and she doesn't remember much about the pregnancy.

Case Study

Today is her first prenatal visit with her midwife. Linda's family doctor had sent her for an ultrasound and she brings the results with her to this appointment. It indicates that the pregnancy is at 14 weeks gestation. Her due date, or estimated date of delivery (EDD), is April 18. Linda has the following concerns: "I am worried about these bumps on my nipples, and why are my breasts so tender? Look at this line on my abdomen; where did that come from? I have this vaginal discharge. It doesn't itch or smell bad, but I notice I am a lot wetter than I have ever been before."

Questions

Respond to Linda's concerns:

1. "I am worried about these bumps on my nipples, and why are my breasts so tender?"

2. "Look at this line on my abdomen; where did that come from and what is the brownish coloring on my face?"

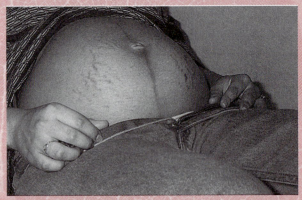

Figure 1.1 *Linea nigra.*

3. "Is it going to always be there?"

4. "I have this vaginal discharge. It doesn't itch or smell bad, but I notice I am a lot wetter than I have ever been before."

5. What is Linda's gravida/para?

6. Linda is very excited because her due date is on her birthday. She asks the nurse how certain it is that the baby will actually be born on that date. How should the nurse respond?

7. Linda admits that maybe she did miss a birth control pill several months ago. She continued to take them up to the day she saw her family doctor about the nausea and vomiting and found out she was pregnant. She asks the nurse how dangerous this might be to the baby she is carrying. How should the nurse reply?

8. Besides ultrasound, how can a due date be identified when there is no regular and accurate menstrual history to rely on?

9. Linda asks the nurse when she can first expect to feel her baby move. What is the best response by the nurse? What is this movement called?

10. Everything is normal at this initial visit. When should the nurse schedule Linda to return for her next prenatal visit?

11. Identify at least three areas of education that the nurse needs to address at this initial visit.

References

Blackburn, S. (2003). *Maternal, fetal and neonatal physiology* (2nd ed.). St Louis: W.B. Saunders Co.

Kuppermann, M., Nease, R. F., Jr., Gates, E., Learman, L. A., Blumberg, B., Gildengorin, V., et al. (2004, June). How do women of diverse backgrounds value prenatal testing outcomes? *Prenat Diagn., 24*(6), 424–429.

Li, De-Kun, Daling, J. R., Mueller, B. A., Hickok, D. E., Fantel, A. G., & Weiss, N. S. (1995). Oral contraceptives use after conception in relation to the risk of congenital urinary tract anomalies. *Teratology, 51,* 30–36.

Wald, N. J., Rodeck, C., Hackshaw, A. K., & Rudnicka, A. (2004, June). SURUSS in perspective. *BJOG: An International Journal of Obstetrics & Gynecology 6,* 521–531.

Wheeler, L. (2002). *Nurse-Midwifery handbook* (2nd ed.). Philadelphia: Lippincott, Williams & Wilkins.

CASE STUDY 2

Aries

AGE

17

SETTING

- Indian Reservation Clinic

CULTURAL CONSIDERATIONS

- Native American traditions

ETHNICITY

- Native American

PRE-EXISTING CONDITION

CO-EXISTING CONDITION/CURRENT PROBLEM

COMMUNICATIONS

DISABILITY

SOCIOECONOMIC STATUS

- Poverty

SPIRITUAL/RELIGIOUS

- Native American traditions

PSYCHOSOCIAL

- No support from fob

LEGAL

ETHICAL

PRIORITIZATION

DELEGATION

PHARMACOLOGIC

- Fe supplementation

ALTERNATIVE THERAPY

SIGNIFICANT HISTORY

- Primigravida

PRENATAL, second trimester

Level of difficulty: Easy

Overview: This case requires an understanding of Native American culture including the influence of the elders and taboos. It also reviews the risks associated with alcohol and tobacco in pregnancy.

7

Client Profile

Aries is a 17-year-old, single, Native American female, G1P0. She is five foot three inches tall and her pre-pregnant weight was 128 pounds. She is single and lives with her mother, two older sisters, and two older brothers in a small home near a reservation. Her father left the family when she was six months old. Her mother has managed to provide for the family by doing housekeeping for one of the wealthy families in town. They think the world of her mother and often give her bonuses to help with her financial problems. Aries and all of her siblings are embarrassed that their mother cleans houses and resent her employer's generosity. Her brothers, although 20 and 21 years old, cannot find work and just hang around the house or get into minor difficulties in town. One of her older sisters is in junior college studying to be a nurse, and the other is a senior in high school. Aries is the youngest and is a high school junior. Aries's grandmother lives nearby and often spends time at the house. It is Aries's grandmother who first brings her to the clinic for prenatal care.

Case Study

This is Aries's first prenatal visit. She had not been using any form of contraception. She did not intend to get pregnant, but did not take seriously the possibility that it could happen to her. Her last normal menstrual period was July 6 (today is November 20). When Aries is asked about her past medical history, the grandmother answers, but only vaguely. Aries is not able to tell the nurse how frequently her periods come. Aries is very respectful of her grandmother and sits quietly without making eye contact with the nurse during the interview. Aries does respond when asked about her use of alcohol and tobacco. She admits to drinking a little on weekends with her friends and smoking about 5 to 6 cigarettes a day. The baby's father boasts about the pregnancy but does not display any indication that he will assume any responsibility for the baby. Recently he has started dating another girl.

Questions

1. If Aries has a 28-day cycle, when is the baby due?

2. How many weeks gestation is she today?

3. What is the possible reason the nurse is having a problem getting a history from Aries and/or her grandmother regarding Aries?

4. What is the significance of Aries's grandmother bringing Aries to the initial prenatal visit?

5. How can the nurse obtain a better estimate of how much Aries drinks?

6. How much weight should Aries gain in the pregnancy?

7. List at least three risk factors associated with Aries's pregnancy.

8. Aries's grandmother instructs her to take herbs to improve her blood, but her sister (a nursing student) wants her to take iron supplements. Which advice do you think Aries will follow? Why?

9. Aries decides to quit school at 20 weeks gestation and stay close to home. She spends more time with her grandmother listening to stories while her grandmother works on quilts and macramé. They do not make anything for the baby. Why?

10. Aries is forbidden from working on the macramé. Why?

11. Give two common mistakes that nurses make when trying to provide care to women from cultures they are not familiar with.

References

Littleton, L., & Engebretson, J. C. (2002). *Maternal, neonatal, and women's health nursing.* Clifton Park, NY: Thomson Delmar Learning.

Simpson, K. R., & Creehan, P. A. (2001). *AWHONN perinatal nursing* (2nd ed.). Philadelphia: Lippincott, Williams & Wilkins.

Fayola

AGE

23

SETTING

- Certified Nurse Midwifery Office

CULTURAL CONSIDERATIONS

- Recent Nigerian immigrant

ETHNICITY

- African

PRE-EXISTING CONDITION

CO-EXISTING CONDITION/CURRENT PROBLEM

- Low back ache at 24 weeks gestational age (wga); r/o PTL; social isolation

COMMUNICATION

- Limited English

DISABILITY

SOCIOECONOMIC STATUS

SPIRITUAL/RELIGIOUS

PSYCHOSOCIAL

- Social isolation

LEGAL

ETHICAL

PRIORITIZATION

DELEGATION

PHARMACOLOGIC

- Tocolytics: ritodrine, terbutaline, magnesium sulfate, indomethacin, nifedipine nicardipine

ALTERNATIVE THERAPY

SIGNIFICANT HISTORY

- Primigravida

PRENATAL

Level of difficulty: Easy

Overview: Requires using critical thinking to identify those pieces of data that either rule in or rule out preterm labor.

Client Profile

Fayola is a 23-year-old G1P0 recent Nigerian immigrant. Her husband is an exchange student at the university doing graduate work in medicine. He works very long hours, leaving her alone most of the time. Her English is not good and she is very shy. She misses her family, especially now that she is pregnant. She started her prenatal care at 8 weeks gestation and looks to her midwife as a replacement mother. This has accounted for at least one phone call a week to the Certified Nurse Midwife (CNM) for one reason or another. Often these calls are just to receive reassurance.

Case Study

Fayola is now 24 wga. She calls the clinic to talk to her midwife with complaints of a low backache.

Questions

1. What are the most common reasons for backaches at 24 wga?

2. List at least five questions the nurse needs to ask Fayola about her backache to begin to assess the necessity of her coming to the clinic at this time.

3. What are Braxton Hicks contractions?

4. Is it common for women expecting their first babies to have uncomfortable Braxton Hicks contractions at this time in their pregnancies?

5. What are the typical characteristics of Braxton Hicks contractions?

6. What advice can the nurse give Fayola if she believes that the contractions are Braxton Hicks?

7. If the nurse suspects preterm labor, what should she advise Fayola to do?

8. Fayola goes to the hospital, where her contractions are timed at being 30 to 40 seconds and coming every 10 minutes. What further evaluation will be done to confirm if these are labor or Braxton Hicks contractions?

9. Fayola has not been drinking much for the past few days. How does dehydration relate to uterine contractions?

10. At the hospital triage Fayola's cervix was found to have no signs of preterm labor. She is given 500 ml of lactated Ringers IV solution, the contractions stop, and after two hours of observation, they discharge her with advice to drink more water on a regular basis. How much should she be drinking and how often?

11. Identify two nursing diagnoses that apply to Fayola at this time.

References

Blackburn, S. (2003). *Maternal, fetal and neonatal physiology* (2nd ed.). St. Louis: W. B. Saunders Co.

Simpson, K. R, & Creehan, P. A. (2001). *AWHONN perinatal nursing* (2nd ed.). Philadelphia: Lippincott, Williams & Wilkins.

Stan, C., Boulvain, M., Hirsbrunner-Amagbaly, P., & Pfister, R. (2003). Hydration for treatment of preterm labour. *The Cochrane Database of Systematic Reviews, 2,* no. CD003096. DOI: 10.1002/14651858.CD003096.

Wheeler, L. (2002). *Nurse-Midwifery handbook* (2nd ed.). Philadelphia: Lippincott, Williams & Wilkins.

Lilly

AGE

36

SETTING

- Birth center

CULTURAL CONSIDERATIONS

- Rural American White culture

ETHNICITY

- White American

PRE-EXISTING CONDITION

- Breastfeeding a toddler while pregnant

CO-EXISTING CONDITION/CURRENT PROBLEM

- AMA; uncertain dates; infectious work environment; exposure to Fifth disease

COMMUNICATIONS

DISABILITY

SOCIOECONOMIC STATUS

SPIRITUAL/RELIGIOUS

PSYCHOSOCIAL

LEGAL

ETHICAL

PRIORITIZATION

- Breastfeeding; family dynamics

DELEGATION

PHARMACOLOGIC

ALTERNATIVE THERAPY

SIGNIFICANT HISTORY

- Multigravida

MODERATE

PRENATAL, second trimester

Level of difficulty: Moderate

Overview: Requires awareness of the risk associated with advanced age in pregnancy, exposure to teratogens, and family dynamics. The student is asked to assess effects of nursing a toddler while pregnant. Establishment of a due date with an unknown LNMP is also explored. This case also asks the student to consider factors that contribute to client satisfaction with the birth experience.

Client Profile

Lilly is a 36-year-old, G2P1001, MWF. Her last child, Katie, is 18 months old and is still nursing at night. Lilly is a certified day care worker in the toddler room at the local YWCA. She loves the job because it means she can be close to her daughter, who is in the room next door. Her husband owns his own landscaping business and enjoys working outdoors. Between them they make a comfortable living. They were just married three years ago and are pleased about this pregnancy since they want several children and feel that they got a late start. Their first daughter was delivered at the birth center. They were both very pleased with her birth and the care they received.

Case Study

Today is Lilly's first prenatal visit to the birth center with this pregnancy. Her husband and daughter accompany her. The nurse finds them in the waiting room going through the center's picture album. They find their picture from their daughter's birth and attempt to get Katie's interest. She briefly looks at it but is more interested in the toys in the children's corner. However, despite Katie's lack of interest, it is clear to the nurse that Lilly and her husband are enjoying reliving the experience through the pictures. After a brief discussion with Lilly and her husband, Lilly goes with the nurse to one of the exam rooms while her husband stays with Katie, who is busy with a set of blocks. The nurse begins Lilly's care by asking for information to establish her due date.

Questions

1. List three questions that the nurse may ask that will help establish Lilly's due date.

2. Lilly states that she first felt the baby move yesterday. If this is so, how far along might Lilly be?

3. As the pregnancy progresses, what other physical signs can be used to help confirm the due date?

4. Why is it important that Lilly's due date be determined during this early visit?

5. Identify two environmental risk factors that could possibly expose Lilly to teratogenic agents.

6. Identify at least two other risk factors for Lilly's pregnancy.

7. Lilly says that she is not ready to completely wean her 18-month-old from the breast. What advice should the nurse give her regarding this?

8. Lilly and her husband have decided that they want their daughter present for the labor and birth. What advice should the nurse offer them regarding this decision?

9. Lilly stated that one of the children at the childcare facility where she works has been diagnosed with Fifth disease. She asks if this is dangerous to her and her baby. How should the nurse respond?

10. What test will be done to determine if Lilly is at risk from Fifth disease?

11. Birth centers do not offer epidurals, and many do not offer any forms of medication for pain relief. Despite this, the level of satisfaction with birth center births is high, often higher than with medicated, hospital births. What factors affect how satisfied a woman is with her birth experience?

References

Biancuzzo, M. (2003). *Breastfeeding the newborn: Clinical strategies for nurses* (2nd ed.). St. Louis: Mosby.

Chang, Mei-Yueh, Wang, Shing-Yaw, & Chen, Chung-Hey. (2002). Effects of massage on pain and anxiety during labour: A randomized controlled trial in Taiwan. *Journal of Advanced Nursing, 38*(1).

Cartter, M. L., Farley, T. A., Rosengren, J., Quinn, D. I., Gillespie, S. M., Gary, G. W., & Hadler,
    J. L. (1991). Occupational risk factors for infection with parvovirus B19 among pregnant
    women. *Journal of Infectious Disease, 163,* 292.

Cunningham, F. G., et al. (2001). *Williams obstetrics* (21st ed.). London: Appleton and Lange.

Himenick, S. (2003, March 4). Post ecstatic birth syndrome. *Vital Signs. 13*(5).

Littleton, L., & Engebretson, J. C. (2002). *Maternal, neonatal, and women's health
    nursing.* Clifton Park, NY: Thomson Delmar Learning.

McCrea, B. H., & Wright, M. E. (1999). Satisfaction in childbirth and perceptions of personal
    control in pain relief during labour. *Journal of Advanced Nursing, 29*(4), 877–884.

Mohrbacher, N., & Stock, J. (2003). *The breastfeeding answer book* (3rd ed.). Schumberg, IL:
    La Leche League International.

Riordan, J., & Auerbach, K. (2005). *Breast feeding and human lactation* (3rd ed.). Sudbury, MA:
    Jones and Bartlett.

Varney, H., Kriebs, J., & Gegor, C. (2004). *Varney's midwifery* (4th ed.). Boston: Jones and
    Bartlett.

Wheeler, L. (2002). *Nurse-Midwifery Handbook* (2nd ed.). Philadelphia: Lippincott, Williams &
    Wilkins.

Florence

AGE

   Adolescent

SETTING

   ■ Prenatal clinic

CULTURAL CONSIDERATIONS

   ■ Rastafarian Jamaican traditions

ETHNICITY

   ■ Jamaican

PRE-EXISTING CONDITION

   ■ Acne; possible teratogenic exposure;
     obesity; possible chronic hypertension

CO-EXISTING CONDITION/CURRENT PROBLEM

   ■ Uncertain dating of pregnancy; hypertension

COMMUNICATIONS

DISABILITY

SOCIOECONOMIC STATUS

SPIRITUAL/RELIGIOUS

   ■ Rastafarian

PSYCHOSOCIAL

   ■ Much older male partner; denial of
     pregnancy; literacy; male dominant/female
     submissive behavior

LEGAL

   ■ Minor (capacity to make decisions related to
     health care); privacy; state laws related to
     reporting statutory rape

ETHICAL

   ■ Self-determination vs client advocacy

PRIORITIZATION

   ■ Need to establish client age and due date;
     establishment of trusting relationship

DELEGATION

PHARMACOLOGIC

   ■ Isotretinoin (Accutane)

ALTERNATIVE THERAPY

SIGNIFICANT HISTORY

PRENATAL

Level of difficulty: Moderate

Overview: Requires an awareness of adolescent behavior, Jamaican culture, and nonverbal communication. Requires awareness of prescription and OTC drug teratogenic potentials.

Client Profile

Florence, a Jamaican teen, presents at the prenatal clinic on August 20. As she registers at the reception desk the nurse begins her assessment by observing that an older male, who appears well groomed and in his late twenties or early thirties, accompanies her. The male companion is the one who fills out the registration information while Florence appears disinterested and casually leafs through a magazine. There doesn't seem to be any verbal exchange between Florence and her companion.

Florence is wearing an oversized sweatshirt and pants. Her hair is pulled back into a ponytail and she is wearing heavy foundation makeup, which may be meant to cover acne. She is wearing an opal pendant around her neck. She is approximately five feet three or four inches tall and the nurse estimates her weight at 160 pounds, although it is a little difficult to be certain with her baggy clothes. Florence continues to turn the pages in an almost automated manner without looking at the print or pictures.

Case Study

The nurse calls Florence's name in the waiting room to have her enter the intake room and begin her interview. As she stands up to follow the nurse, her companion also stands and begins to follow her. Florence seems to expect this. The nurse stops and explains that initially she always interviews new clients alone, but she respects his desire to be involved and will call him in later. At first both Florence and her companion are taken aback by this arrangement; however, the nurse's matter-of-fact approach and her warm manner and willingness to involve him "as soon as possible" put them both off guard and Florence follows the nurse alone.

The following additional data is collected:

FH 26 cm

Urine dip indicated negative protein, glucose; positive ketones, nitrites, and leukocytes

BP 138/84

Actual weight is 168 pounds (She states that her prepregnant weight was around 158 to 160 pounds.)

An ultrasound is done and it is determined that Florence is approximately 26 weeks gestation at this initial visit.

Questions

1. Discuss the significance of Florence's appearance and behavior.

2. Discuss the significance of the companion's behaviors.

3. Which of the following do you believe was the rationale for the nurse's behavior?

  a. She was establishing her authority in the clinic setting.

  b. She was protecting Florence's privacy during the health interview.

  c. She was letting the "man" know that, although he wishes to be involved, there will be a time and a place for his involvement.

  d. She desired to hear how Florence would answer questions, not how her companion would answer them for her.

4. During the interview Florence states that her last menstrual period was March 16. What is Florence's due date?

5. What questions need to be answered to determine how accurate this due date is?

6. What are the implications of her coming so late for prenatal care?

7. Nutrition is always important during pregnancy. State two reasons the nurse needs to be especially concerned about this client's nutritional habits.

8. Florence is covering her acne with a heavy makeup foundation. Some acne medications are known to be teratogenic. Which ones are dangerous, and when are they the most dangerous? What advice can the nurse give Florence regarding treatment for her acne during pregnancy?

9. What is the significance of the positive ketones in her urine?

10. What is the implication of the positive nitrites and leukocytes esterase in the urine?

11. Florence tells the nurse that her usual blood pressure is 118–120/65–75. Describe the normal blood pressure changes in pregnancy. Does Florence's blood pressure at this initial visit fit into the normal pattern expected for this time in her pregnancy?

References

Blackburn, S. (2003). *Maternal, fetal and neonatal physiology* (2nd ed.). St. Louis; W.B. Saunders Co.

Littleton, L., & Engebretson, J. C. (2002). *Maternal, neonatal, and women's health nursing.* Clifton Park, NY: Thomson Delmar Learning.

Littleton, L., & Engebretson, J. C. (2005). *Maternity nursing care.* Clifton Park, NY: Thomson Delmar Learning.

Simpson, K. R., & Creehan, P. A. (2001). *AWHONN perinatal nursing* (2nd ed.). Philadelphia: Lippincott, Williams & Wilkins.

Ruby

AGE

43

SETTING

- Women's clinic

CULTURAL CONSIDERATIONS

- White middle-class American culture

ETHNICITY

- White American

PRE-EXISTING CONDITION

- Obesity

CO-EXISTING CONDITION/CURRENT PROBLEM

- AMA; perimenopausal; 2nd trimester spotting; high fundal height; hepatitis B vaccine; severe N&V

COMMUNICATIONS

DISABILITY

SOCIOECONOMIC STATUS

SPIRITUAL/RELIGIOUS

PSYCHOSOCIAL

LEGAL

ETHICAL

PRIORITIZATION

DELEGATION

PHARMACOLOGIC

ALTERNATIVE THERAPY

SIGNIFICANT HISTORY

- Multigravida

MODERATE

ANTEPARTUM

Level of difficulty: Moderate

Overview: In the case the student is asked to assess perimenopausal symptoms and an unplanned AMA pregnancy as well as explores causes of early pregnancy spotting. This case also looks at vaccination during pregnancy.

Client Profile

Ruby is a 43-year-old, G4P2103, divorced White American female. Her youngest child is now 23 years old. Ruby is an art teacher at a local junior high school. She has been having unusually heavy, irregular periods for approximately six months, and then no period for the past three months. During these three months she has been very fatigued and experiencing nausea and vomiting twice a day. Ruby is five feet four inches tall, and her current weight is 140 pounds. Despite the nausea and vomiting, she has gained five pounds in the past three months.

Case Study

Ruby came to the women's clinic today to get information on menopause and to find out why she has been feeling so sick. A pregnancy test came back positive. Her physical exam confirmed a uterus enlarged to a 16 weeks size and FHTs were heard. Ruby is spotting. She just finished a series of injections of the hepatitis B vaccine. Ruby is in mild disbelief!

Questions

1. What is the most probable cause of her heavy irregular periods in the years just prior to the menopause?

2. What are the risks associated with this pregnancy?

3. What screening tests are available to screen for congenital anomalies?

4. What is Ruby's BMI? How much weight should Ruby gain?

5. List at least five common signs and symptoms of menopause.

6. When can a woman consider herself in menopause and therefore discontinue birth control?

7. What information can the nurse use to try to determine Ruby's due date?

8. Give four possible reasons for Ruby's spotting.

9. Ruby's fundal height is high for the dates she reports. Name two possible reasons for this, and explain your answers.

10. Are there risks associated with hepatitis B vaccine during pregnancy?

References

Blackburn, S. (2003). *Maternal, fetal, and neonatal physiology* (2nd ed.). St. Louis, MO: W.B. Saunders Co.

NAMS Professional Education Committee. (2004). *Menopause practice: a clinician's guide.* Cleveland, OH: North American Menopause Society.

Varney, H., Kriebs, J., & Gegor, C. (2004). *Varney's midwifery* (4th ed.). Boston: Jones and Bartlett.

Caridad

AGE

26

SETTING

- Prenatal clinic

CULTURAL CONSIDERATIONS

- Caribbean culture

ETHNICITY

- Hispanic American

PRE-EXISTING CONDITION

CO-EXISTING CONDITION/CURRENT PROBLEM

- No fetal movement in 24 hours; fetal demise; tobacco use

COMMUNICATIONS

DISABILITY

SOCIOECONOMIC STATUS

SPIRITUAL/RELIGIOUS

PSYCHOSOCIAL

LEGAL

ETHICAL

PRIORITIZATION

DELEGATION

PHARMACOLOGIC

- Oxytocin (Pitocin)

ALTERNATIVE THERAPY

SIGNIFICANT HISTORY

- Primigravida

MODERATE

PRENATAL/INTRAPARTUM

Level of difficulty: Moderate

Overview: Requires using critical thinking to assess and care for a woman who has experienced an intrauterine fetal loss.

Client Profile   **Caridad** is a 26-year-old, G1P0, MHF at 28 wga. Her pregnancy thus far has been uneventful except for some spotting during the first six weeks. Caridad smokes 3 to 4 cigarettes a day.

Case Study   Caridad calls the prenatal clinic to say that earlier this morning she had felt her baby move a lot. She said the movement was so violent that it actually hurt her. Now she realizes that she has not felt her baby move again all day. She is told to come in, and the baby's heart tones are checked. They cannot be located. An ultrasound is ordered, and the diagnosis of fetal demise is made.

Questions

1. Is there a relationship between the spotting during the first trimester and later intrauterine fetal death (IUFD)?

2. Caridad is not experiencing any bleeding or cramping at this time. What is the probability that she will go into spontaneous labor soon?

3. If she does not go into labor, how will the pregnancy be terminated?

4. What are the risks for Caridad if she decides to wait for her body to naturally go into labor?

5. What lab work should the nurse anticipate for Caridad?

6. What emotional and/or psychological responses should the nurse anticipate from Caridad during her labor?

7. How might this experience affect Caridad in future pregnancies?

8. How might the nurse guide Caridad's family to support her during this time?

9. How likely is it that her smoking caused the fatal demise?

10. After two weeks it is determined that Caridad needs to be induced. Her cervix is still long and closed, firm and midline. Describe how prostaglandins can be used to prepare the cervix for induction. Include nursing responsibilities related to safety during this procedure.

References

Panuthos, C., & Romeo, C. (1984). *Ended beginnings.* South Hadley, MA: Bergin & Garvey Publishers, Inc.

Varney, H., Kriebs, J., & Gegor, C. (2004). *Varney's midwifery* (4th ed.). Boston: Jones and Bartlett.

Esparanza

AGE

23

SETTING

- Private prenatal office

CULTURAL CONSIDERATIONS

- Mexican traditional health beliefs

ETHNICITY

- Hispanic American

PRE-EXISTING CONDITION

- Previous breech birth

CO-EXISTING CONDITION/CURRENT PROBLEM

- Breech presentation

COMMUNICATIONS

DISABILITY

SOCIOECONOMIC STATUS

SPIRITUAL/RELIGIOUS

PSYCHOSOCIAL

LEGAL

ETHICAL

- Client needs vs practitioner's needs

PRIORITIZATION

- Safety vs client desire for VBAC

DELEGATION

PHARMACOLOGIC

- RhoGAM

ALTERNATIVE THERAPY

- Moxibustion; light; music

SIGNIFICANT HISTORY

- Multigravida; previous cesarean section

PRENATAL

Level of difficulty: Difficult

Overview: Requires knowledge regarding breech presentations and cesarean section. This case asks students to use critical thinking to compare and contrast VBAC and cesarean section and the types of anesthesia used.

DIFFICULT

Client Profile

Esparanza is a 23-year-old, G2P1001, MHF at 36 wga. She had a previous cesarean section with an epidural in Mexico six years ago for a breech presentation at 38 weeks gestational age. The baby weighed six pounds. She is five feet two inches tall, and her PPW was 100 pounds. She would like a vaginal birth after cesarean section (VBAC) with this pregnancy, however she saw six doctors before she found one who would even consider doing a VBAC.

Case Study

Esparanza seems anxious at today's prenatal visit. She tells the nurse that the baby feels like his head is up under her ribs and she fears another cesarean section for breech. The following data is obtained at this visit:

Wt 125 lb

FHT 140s URQ

Fundal height (FH) 35 cm

Fetal movement +(FM)

Urine chemstrip testing: all negative

No HA, vision changes

No CVAT

No edema

Questions

1. Why was it so difficult for Esparanza to find an obstetrician who would consider doing a VBAC? Discuss the ethical dilemmas that exist when the desires and needs of the client come in conflict with those of the practitioner.

2. What are the routine labs for this visit, and why are they done at this time?

3. Compare and contrast VBAC and repeat cesarean section for the following: safety for both mother and baby, cost, pain; long-term effects, effects on breastfeeding, and parenting.

4. Her obstetrician asks for her previous cesarean section records before he will even consider a VBAC. Why?

5. Why are cesarean sections usually done for breech presentation?

6. When would a vaginal delivery be considered for a breech presentation?

7. How can the baby be encouraged to move to a cephalic presentation?

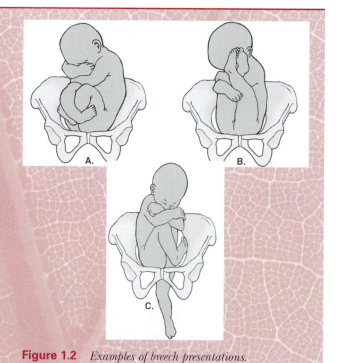

Figure 1.2 *Examples of breech presentations.*

8. What maternal/fetal conditions contribute to a baby presenting in a breech presentation?

9. Compare and contrast spinal and epidural anesthesia for cesarean section.

10. If the baby changes to a cephalic presentation in the next two weeks but Esparanza does not go into spontaneous labor, can she be safely induced for a VBAC?

11. What methods can be used if any?

12. Esparanza begins to cry at the 39-week visit when she realizes that the baby has not yet changed position. She says that "I just know it's going to be terrible again. I'll never be able to breastfeed my baby postpartum; it's so painful." How should the nurse respond?

References

Biancuzzo, M. (2003). *Breastfeeding the newborn: Clinical strategies for nurses* (2nd ed.). St Louis, MO: Mosby.

Littleton, L., & Engebretson, J. C. (2002). *Maternal, neonatal, and women's health nursing.* Clifton Park, NY: Thomson Delmar Learning.

Riordan, J., & Auerbach, K. (2005). *Breast feeding and human lactation* (3rd ed.). Sudbury, MA: Jones and Bartlett.

Simpson, K. R., & Creehan P. A. (2001). *AWHONN perinatal nursing* (2nd ed.). Philadelphia: Lippincott, Williams & Wilkins.

Tiran, D., & Mack, S. (2000). *Complementary therapies for pregnancy and childbirth* (2nd ed.). London: Baillière Tindall.

Sarah

AGE

36

SETTING

- Free clinic

CULTURAL CONSIDERATIONS

ETHNICITY

- White American

PRE-EXISTING CONDITION

CO-EXISTING CONDITION/CURRENT PROBLEM

- Uncertain EDC; financial problems; yeast infection

COMMUNICATIONS

DISABILITY

SOCIOECONOMIC STATUS

- Low income (no health insurance)

SPIRITUAL/RELIGIOUS

PSYCHOSOCIAL

LEGAL

ETHICAL

- Need for care vs ability to pay

PRIORITIZATION

DELEGATION

PHARMACOLOGIC

ALTERNATIVE THERAPY

SIGNIFICANT HISTORY

- Adopted; history of pregnancy loss— 2 spontaneous abortions, 1 preterm loss; mulitgravida

PRENATAL

Level of difficulty: Difficult

Overview: Requires identification of history strongly suggestive of diabetes. Requires critical thinking to set priorities for care. Ask students to consider social responsibility concerns.

Client Profile

Sarah is a 36-year-old, G4P0120, MWF at approximately 18 weeks gestation at her initial PNV (according to unsure dates and uterine size). She presents to a reduced fee clinic run by the Kiwanis Club. She is five feet three inches and her pre-pregnant weight was 136 pounds.

Case Study

Her chief complaints at this visit include positive pregnancy test five weeks ago, vaginal discharge (white cheesy odorless), and pruritus. Her medical history includes recurrent urinary tract infections and yeast infections. She has a negative surgical history. She was adopted and does not know her family history. Significant OB history includes two spontaneous abortions (SAB). One was three years ago at 12 weeks and one was six months ago at 10 to 12 weeks. She also had a loss of a 32-week infant following complications associated with preterm premature rupture of membranes (PPROM) two years ago. The infant weighed 8 pounds and died from respiratory distress syndrome (RDS) and sepsis (early onset GBS). The baby lived 14 hours and also experienced jaundice, hypoglycemia, temperature instability, and acidosis.

Sarah and her husband both work two part-time jobs each. They have no health insurance and earn too much for Medicaid. Although they manage to pay their bills, there is seldom anything left for health care. Subsequently, neither one is able to receive regular checkups. As a matter of fact, the last time Sarah saw a doctor was when she went into labor with her preterm baby two years ago. (She was not receiving prenatal care for that pregnancy.) When she had her last SAB she bled for about two months but did not seek medical care. She felt that she had been through this before and that it would stop on its own. It did, and she resumed work after several weeks. They are still paying for her last hospitalization and the bills for the baby they lost. This accounts for why she waited until 18 weeks to seek prenatal care at this time. She might have waited longer except that a friend told her about the Kiwanis clinic and suggested that she might be able to afford care there.

Today she tells you that, although they have the money for the $20 office visit, they only have enough money to pay for some of the lab work. This couple does not want to return to the county hospital because they do not qualify for any financial relief, and the cost of care for those who have to pay at the county hospital is very high. The only advantages the county hospital holds for them are that they can receive care (will not be turned away) and they can make small payments. They already feel that they will spend the rest of their lives trying to pay off the preterm baby they lost, and they do not wish to add to their debt for this pregnancy. Like many couples they "slip through the cracks" in our medical system and have little choice for care. They ask the nurse what lab tests they *really need* to have done at this time and which ones can wait until they can bring in more money.

Questions

1. Based on Sarah's obstetrical history, list two major concerns for this pregnancy.

2. Review what is included in initial prenatal lab work. She is already approximately 18 weeks. What lab work is crucial for her at this time, and what can safely wait?

3. What other sources might you direct this couple to for financial help?

4. Can you predict any prenatal complications from the data previously given?

5. If this couple lived in your hometown, what would be the options open to them for care?

6. Discuss the following statement: "Not providing adequate prenatal care is much more expensive than providing it."

7. If you were in a political position to change the health care system regarding maternity care, how would you change it?

8. As a student, what can you do to bring situations like this to the forefront so that individuals who have the power to change things will respond?

9. Discuss your professional responsibility to become involved in policy decision making regarding availability of medical care.

10. Free clinics (those that only charge the exact cost of supplies used) or reduced-cost clinics are sometimes able to provide care at much lower fees than mainstream care facilities. Sometimes free clinics are subsidized to be able to provide care at no cost. One reason they can do that is volunteer professional help. In the past, charitable facilities were protected from lawsuits by sovereign immunity. This protection has been removed in many areas. What is the status in your area? How does having, or not having, sovereign immunity affect the cost of health care? Discuss the pros and cons of these legal changes.

References

Littleton, L., & Engebretson, J. C. (2002). *Maternal, neonatal, and women's health nursing.* Clifton Park, NY: Thomson Delmar Learning.

Rostant, D. M., & Cady, R. (1999). *AWHONN liability issues in perinatal nursing.* Philadelphia: Lippincott, Williams & Wilkins.

Wheeler, L. (2002). *Nurse-midwifery handbook* (2nd ed.). Philadelphia: Lippincott, Williams & Wilkins.

Kathie

AGE

16

SETTING

- Prenatal clinic

CULTURAL CONSIDERATIONS

ETHNICITY

- White American

PRE-EXISTING CONDITION

CO-EXISTING CONDITION/CURRENT PROBLEM

- UTI/kidney; BV; HPV; severe N&V with weight loss; uncertain due date

COMMUNICATIONS

- Third-grade reading level

DISABILITY

SOCIOECONOMIC STATUS

- Lives with grandmother in subsidized housing; poverty

SPIRITUAL/RELIGIOUS

PSYCHOSOCIAL

- Third-grade educational level; unrealistic expectations; fob is married

LEGAL

- Statutory rape

ETHICAL

PRIORITIZATION

- Need to establish client age and due date; establishment of trusting relationship

DELEGATION

PHARMACOLOGIC

ALTERNATIVE THERAPY

SIGNIFICANT HISTORY

- Primigravida

PRENATAL

Level of difficulty: Difficult

Overview: Requires that the nurse understand some of the misconceptions common among teens with low literacy levels regarding their sexuality, fantasy thinking, and health problems often related to these misconceptions and unsafe behaviors.

Client Profile

Kathie is a 16-year-old, SWF who has missed four periods. She lives with her grandmother. The grandmother raised her and her two sisters. Kathie is the youngest. One of her sisters has two children. They all live together in a three-bedroom, subsidized apartment. Kathie is five feet six inches, and her current weight is 110 lbs. As far as she can remember, her pre-pregnant weight was 108. She states that the fob, a 28-year-old married man, denies this is his baby. Kathie states that she is not worried, that he will "come around and love this baby." Kathie attends an overcrowded, inner-city high school and is a junior. She can neither read nor write above the third-grade level. She tells the midwife that when she graduates she wants to become a doctor.

Case Study

Kathie can't believe that she is pregnant since she had been douching for birth control every time she had intercourse. She complains of excessive vomiting and states that she has lost 10 pounds in the past two weeks. Other complaints include intermittent chills, pain in the lower right back area, and pain with voiding. She has dark circles under her eyes and her mucus membranes are dry and pale. Her vital signs are: BP 108/68, T 103.8°F, P 88, and R 22.

Upon examining the midwife notes:

1. Right side, cervical lymph glands are enlarged and tender
2. Needs dental work on two of her upper right molars
3. Fundal height is three fingers below the umbilicus
4. FHT are heard in the LLQ (130s)
5. When doing her PAP the midwife notes that she has a homogenous gray clinging discharge with a pH of 5.5
6. The wet mount has clue cells (epithelial cells with a stippled appearance)
7. The whiff test (a fishy odor when potassium hydroxide is added to the vaginal secretions) is also positive
8. Wart-like growths on the outside of her vagina with positive ascetic-white test
9. Urine chemstrip in the office is positive for ketones, nitrites, and leukocytes; negative for glucose and protein.

Kathie is given HIV counseling and agrees to be tested. Her HIV test comes back negative.

Questions

1. If Kathie's size equals her dates, about how many weeks pregnant do you think she is?

2. Why do you think she put off coming in for prenatal care so long?

3. How important is it that her due date be established at this first visit?

4. In light of Kathie's advanced gestation and weight loss, how significant is her nausea and vomiting?

5. Which of Kathie's signs and symptoms point to a urinary tract infection? How serious are these signs and symptoms?

6. What are the implications of UTI for pregnancy?

7. What is the significance of the homogenous gray clinging discharge, positive whiff test, and finding of the clue cells?

8. What are vaginal warts that turn white with ascetic acid probably caused by?

9. What is the most likely reason Kathie has swollen cervical lymph glands?

10. What are the implications of dental caries/infections for pregnancy?

11. Discuss common misconceptions teens have about contraception.

12. Make a list of topics the nurse should discuss with Kathie as a result of the initial exam.

13. Make a list of topics to be discussed with Kathie regarding a healthy pregnancy.

14. In light of Kathie's reading level, how will the nurse provide education?

References

Blackburn, S. (2003). *Maternal, fetal & neonatal physiology* (2nd ed.). St. Louis: W.B. Saunders Co.

Freda, M. (2002). *Perinatal patient education*. Philadelphia: Lippincott, Williams & Wilkins.

Littleton, L., & Engebretson, J. C. (2002). *Maternal, neonatal, and women's health nursing*. Clifton Park, NY: Thomson Delmar Learning.

Morgan, G., & Hamilton, C. (2003). *Practice guidelines for obstetrics and gynecology* (2nd ed.). Philadelphia: Lippincott, Williams & Wilkins.

Simpson, K. R., & Creehan, P. A. (2001). *AWHONN Perinatal Nursing* (2nd ed.). Philadelphia: Lippincott, Williams & Wilkins.

Wheeler, L. (2002). *Nurse-Midwifery handbook* (2nd ed.). Philadelphia: Lippincott, Williams & Wilkins.

Whitneye, N., Cataldo, C. B., and Rolfer, S. R. (2002). *Understanding normal and clinical nutrition*. Belmont, CA: Thompson/Wadsworth Learning.

Ruth

AGE	**SPIRITUAL/RELIGIOUS**
28	■ Traditional Native American spiritual beliefs
SETTING	**PSYCHOSOCIAL**
■ Birth center prenatal clinic	
CULTURAL CONSIDERATIONS	**LEGAL**
■ Native American traditions	
ETHNICITY	**ETHICAL**
■ Native American	
PRE-EXISTING CONDITION	**PRIORITIZATION**
■ Asthma; obesity	
CO-EXISTING CONDITION/CURRENT PROBLEM	**DELEGATION**
■ Late entry into care; multiple gestation; blurred vision; tobacco use	**PHARMACOLOGIC**
COMMUNICATIONS	■ Hemabate; methylergonovine maleate (Methergine); oxytocin (Pitocin)
	ALTERNATIVE THERAPY
DISABILITY	
	SIGNIFICANT HISTORY
SOCIOECONOMIC STATUS	■ Grand multigravida; history of preterm births; history of infant losses; history of postpartum hemorrhage
■ Lower middle class	

PRENATAL

Level of difficulty: Difficult

Overview: Requires background knowledge of the Native American culture and health concerns. Requires knowledge regarding asthma and asthma medications and their effects during pregnancy.

Client Profile

Ruth is a 28-year-old, married Native American, G5P2202. Ruth is a social worker on an Indian reservation in North Carolina. Her husband manages a large construction company. Her first two pregnancies occurred when she was a single teen and ended in premature births of infants at 26 and 28 weeks gestation. Both babies died from respiratory distress syndrome (RDS). Ruth was 15 years old with her first baby and 17 with the second. Ruth smoked 1 to 2 packs of cigarettes a day with her first pregnancies and did not start prenatal care until the second trimester with both of them. She was married at age 21 and had two full term pregnancies. The second two children are now one and five years old. They were both NSVD at the small birth center near the reservation. Because of Ruth's job she is well known and loved by everyone in the area. Ruth and her husband, also a Native American, are very proud of their heritage and love living near the reservation, which allows them to keep their children immersed in their culture. Ruth's grandmother is a story-teller for the tribe, and the grandchildren look forward to spending Saturday evenings with her listening to tales about Indian children. Because Ruth's work keeps her so busy she has put off starting her prenatal care for this pregnancy for several months. Although Ruth still smokes one-half pack of cigarettes a day and is overweight, she has been careful to eat properly and get adequate rest when she can.

Case Study

Today (August 15) is her initial prenatal visit at the birth center. Her last normal menstrual period (LNMP) was March 10, and she experienced some spotting on April 2. Ruth has had one minor bout of asthma since getting pregnant. (She uses an inhaler once or twice a week.) Her height is five feet two inches, and her current weight is 186 pounds. She has gained approximately 42 pounds during this pregnancy, so far. Upon examination the nurse finds her fundal height to be 29 cm. Her BP is 112/68, H&H 11.2 mg and 34%. Ruth states that this baby is very active. She has some dependent edema in both ankles. She has not experienced any headaches. She did state that her glasses don't seem to properly correct her vision these days, and the words are sometimes unclear when she tries to read. She is still experiencing some nausea and vomiting, but it is not severe. A wet mount at this visit reveals that Ruth has a vaginal candidiasis (yeast) infection. The routine labs are drawn and cultures done.

Questions

1. How many weeks gestation is Ruth at this initial visit?

2. Identify at least six high-risk factors that Ruth is presenting with.

3. Discuss Ruth's vision changes.

4. Native Americans have a higher risk for diabetes. Does Ruth present any indications of this problem?

5. During the antepartum, culture may influence what taboos and what prescriptives are needed to ensure a safe delivery (Littleton, 2001). When caring for individuals of the Native American culture the nurse should know some of the basic beliefs and behaviors that are practiced in this culture. Name four major areas where misunderstanding can occur between the non–Native American nurse and the Native American family.

6. Native Americans have higher poverty and unemployment rates than other groups of Americans. How does this affect the general health care and outcomes for Native American women?

7. Aside from diabetes, what else could account for her high fundal height?

8. Asthma is also more prevalent in the Native American population. Identify the risk associated with asthma in pregnancy.

9. Overall, how do the statistics on the Native American population compare for preterm births and teen pregnancies to other populations living in the same areas.

10. An ultrasound reveals that Ruth is carrying twins. Make a list of risks that are associated with multiple gestation pregnancies.

11. Ruth goes into preterm labor at 32 weeks gestation and delivers twin boys weighing in at 3 pounds and 2 pounds 6 ounces in the hospital. Immediately following delivery of the placenta she begins to hemorrhage. Her uterus is boggy, and the obstetrician calls for carboprost tromethamine (Hemabate) stat, while he does a bimanual compression. Is this an appropriate order for this client?

12. What would have been the immediate response if the nurse had prepared the medication and the physician had given it?

13. Name two other medications that can be used for this client that will contract the uterus.

14. List and explain at least four factors that placed Ruth at risk for this hemorrhage.

References

Cunningham, F. G., et al. (1993). *Williams Obstetrics* (19th ed.). Norwalk, CT: Appleton & Lange.

Office for Minority Health and Center for Health statistics. *North Carolina Minority Health Facts: Native Americans* (1999).

Simpson, K. R, & Creehan, P. A. (2001). *AWHONN perinatal nursing* (2nd ed.). Philadelphia: Lippincott, Williams & Wilkins.

Garwick, A. (2000). What do providers need to know about Native American culture? Recommendations from urban Indian family caregivers. *Families, Systems & Health: The Journal of Collaborative Family HealthCare, 18*(2).

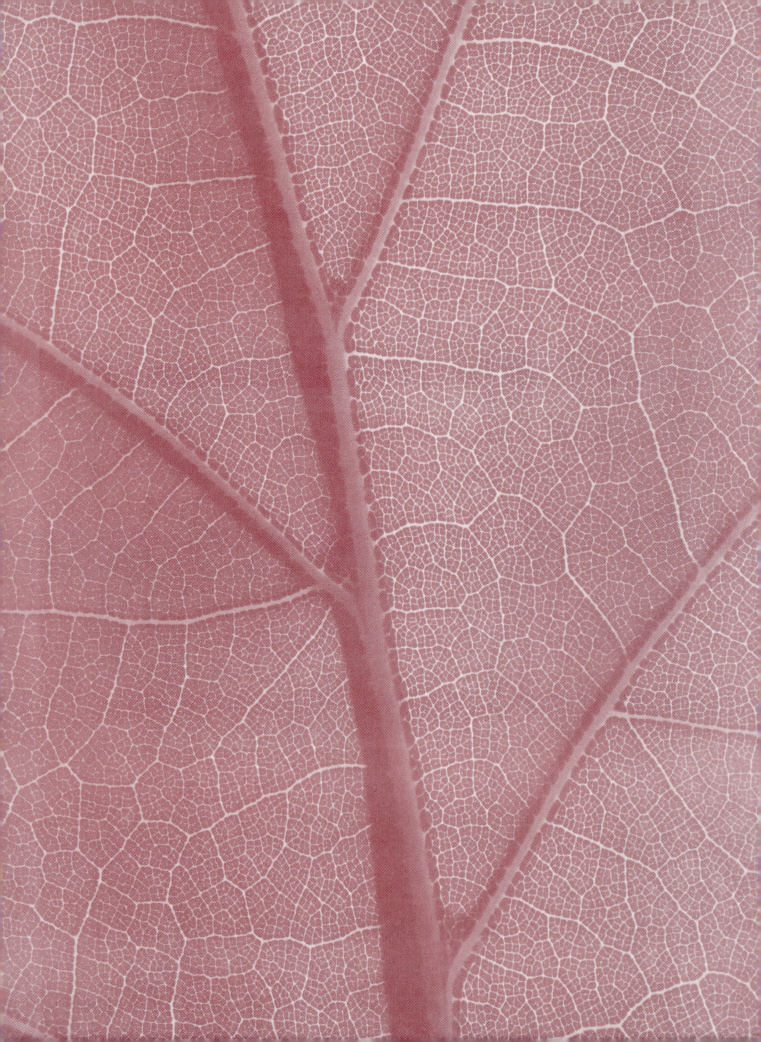

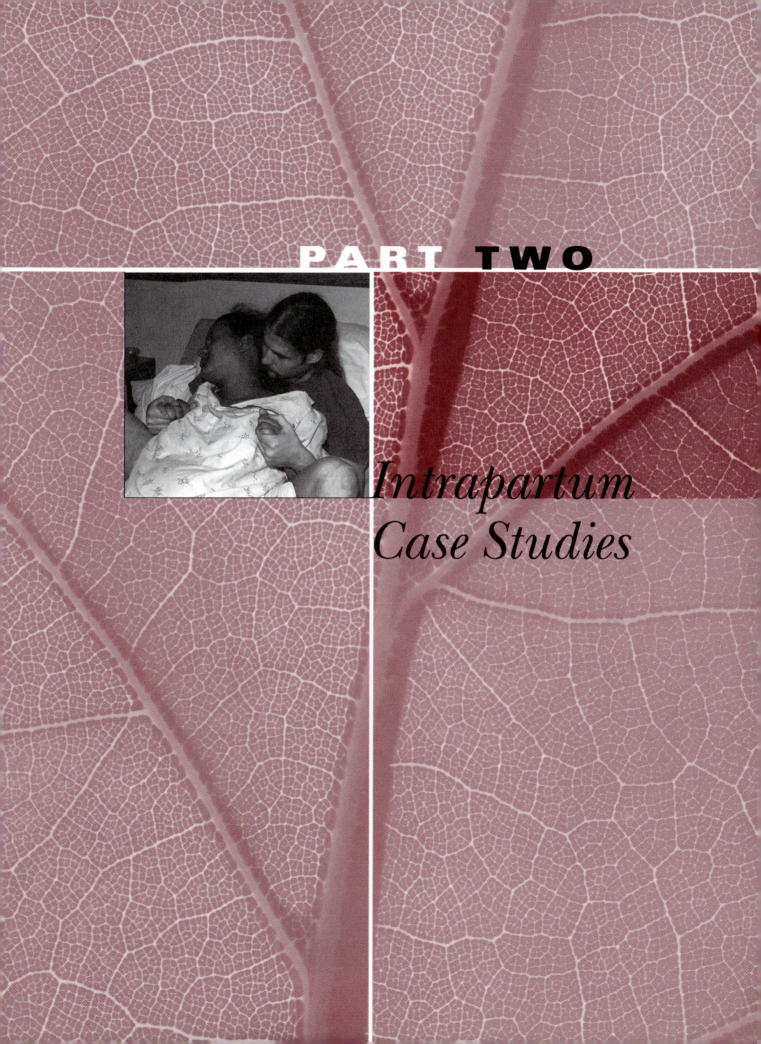

PART TWO

Intrapartum
Case Studies

Norma

AGE

19

SETTING

- Certified Nurse Midwifery office/phone triage

CULTURAL CONSIDERATIONS

- Middle-class White American culture

ETHNICITY

- White American

PRE-EXISTING CONDITION

CO-EXISTING CONDITION/CURRENT PROBLEMS

COMMUNICATIONS

DISABILITY

SOCIOECONOMIC STATUS

SPIRITUAL/RELIGIOUS

PSYCHOSOCIAL

LEGAL

ETHICAL

PRIORITIZATION

DELEGATION

PHARMACOLOGIC

ALTERNATIVE THERAPY

- Aromatherapy: clary sage, jasmine, lavender, nutmeg, rose, ylang-ylang; massage

SIGNIFICANT HISTORY

- Primigravida

INTRAPARTUM

Level of difficulty: Easy

Overview: This case requires an understanding of early labor and asks the student to use critical thinking to assess contractions and fetal well-being.

Client Profile

Norma is a 19-year-old, G1P0, MWF at 39 weeks gestation. Her pregnancy has been uneventful. Norma prides herself on having taken very good care of herself during the pregnancy. Norma is five feet three inches tall and weighs 138 pounds, having gained 22 pounds during the pregnancy.

Case Study

Norma calls her midwife's office to tell her that she has been having contractions for several hours. She tells the nurse that the baby is active, and although she cannot really rest because of the contractions, she feels she is doing very well. Norma has planned a hospital delivery with a certified nurse midwife (CNM).

Questions

1. List three questions the nurse should ask Norma at this time.

2. When should Norma be instructed to go to the hospital?

3. Norma has attended childbirth education classes. She plans to use aromatherapy, water, and massage for pain relief. How effective are these modalities in providing pain relief in labor?

4. Norma has also discussed with the certified nurse midwife (CNM) the use of intermittent fetal monitoring. Discuss the pros and cons of using continuous electronic fetal monitoring in labor.

5. Norma has also asked that she be allowed to not have an IV in labor. Her CNM has agreed to this. Discuss the pros and cons of routine IV in labor.

6. Furthermore, Norma has asked to be able to eat lightly and drink high-energy liquids in labor. Discuss the pros and cons of this.

7. Several hours later, Norma again calls the office to say that she feels she should go to the hospital. Her contractions are coming every three minutes and are lasting from one minute to 90 seconds. When she arrives at the hospital she is found to be 6 cm dilatated, completely effaced, and the baby is a +1 station. Her membranes are intact. The CNM gives her the option of having her membranes ruptured at this time (Figure 2.1). Discuss the pros and cons of this intervention.

8. The nurse is checking the fetus and Norma's contractions intermittently. How often should they be assessed?

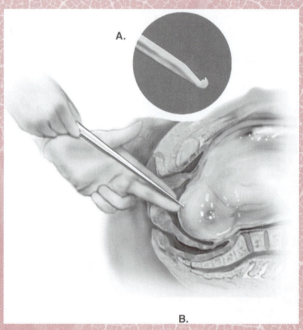

Figure 2.1 *Artificial rupture of membranes (AROM).*

9. How are contractions assessed in labor?

10. After two hours of continued strong contractions Norma is completely effaced and 10 cm dilatated. Norma says she is tired, doesn't feel like pushing, and wants to rest prior to pushing. Discuss the pros and cons of allowing her to rest at this time.

References

Blackburn, S. (2003). *Maternal, fetal, and neonatal physiology* (2nd ed.). St. Louis, MO: W. B. Saunders Co.

Enkin, M., Keirse, M., Neilson, J., Crowther, C., Duley, L. E., et al. (2000). *A guide to an effective care in pregnancy and childbirth.* New York: Oxford University Press.

Feinstein, N. F., Sprague, A., & Trepanier, M. J. (2000). *Fetal heart rate auscultation.* Washington, DC: Association of Women's Health, Obstetric and Neonatal Nurses (AWHONN).

Kubli, M., Scrutton, M. J., Seed, P. T., & O'Sullivan, G. (2002). An evaluation of isotonic "sports drinks" during labor. *Anesthesia & Analgesia, 94*(2), 404–408.

Nichols, F. & Humenick, S. (2000). *Childbirth education practice, research and theory* (2nd ed.). Philadelphia: W. B. Saunders Co.

Varney, H., Kriebs, J., & Gegor, C. (2004). *Varney's midwifery* (4th ed.). Boston: Jones and Bartlett.

Walsh, L. (2001). *Midwifery: community-based care during the childbearing year.* Philadelphia: W. B. Saunders Co.

Holly

AGE

29

SETTING

■ Home

CULTURAL CONSIDERATIONS

ETHNICITY

■ White American

PRE-EXISTING CONDITION

■ Blindness

CO-EXISTING CONDITION/CURRENT PROBLEMS

■ Postdate

COMMUNICATIONS

■ Client is blind

DISABILITY

■ Blindness

SOCIOECONOMIC STATUS

■ Upper middle class

SPIRITUAL/RELIGIOUS

PSYCHOSOCIAL

■ Extended family support

LEGAL

ETHICAL

PRIORITIZATION

DELEGATION

PHARMACOLOGIC

ALTERNATIVE THERAPY

SIGNIFICANT HISTORY

■ Primigravida; auto accident causing blindness

INTRAPARTUM

Level of difficulty: Easy

Overview: This case looks at the difference between a post-date and a post-mature fetus. It explores the advantage of home birth for a client with sensory deprivation, i.e., a blind client.

Client Profile

Holly is a 29-year-old, blind, G1P0, MWF at 41 weeks gestation. Holly is an attorney for the state family and children's division and is now on maternity leave. Holly lost her sight 13 years ago as a result of a head injury in an auto accident. She is an extremely determined individual and finished high school after her accident, went on to a community college, became a paralegal, got her criminal justice degree, and finally completed law school. It took her a little longer than most individuals but she graduated with honors. She met her husband in law school and they have been happily married for two years. She did her internship at the Division of Children and Families for the state and they were so impressed by her abilities that they hired her right after graduation. Holly's 14-year-old sister moved in with her two years ago. Both of their parents were killed in the accident that blinded Holly. Until two years ago her sister had been living with an aunt. She and her sister are very close, and the sister cannot wait until the baby is born so she can help care for him. Holly's pregnancy has progressed normally. All of her lab work is wnl. The baby is in a cephalic presentation. Last week Holly's midwife ordered a NST, which was reactive. Holly has also been doing daily fetal movement counts, and they have demonstrated an active healthy baby.

Case Study

Holly is in active labor at home at 41-2/7 weeks gestation. She wants a home birth since she feels that she will be in familiar surroundings and feel more in control. Two midwives have been with Holly for the past three hours monitoring her baby and contractions. She is now 8 cm, 100% effaced, and +1 station. Holly's husband and sister have been wonderful support for her. During the contractions they take turns dancing with Holly, and even though she is in transition she responds positively to their support and gets relief by the movement. The baby's heart rate is in the 140s with good long-term variability. There are no decelerations, and there are occasional accelerations. Holly's water breaks with a large gush. The fluid is clear without any odor.

Questions

1. What are the advantages for Holly in a home birth?

2. What coping mechanisms is Holly using to deal with the contractions? Why are these particularly good for Holly?

3. In general, discuss the safety of a planned home birth.

4. Why did the midwife order a non-stress test (NST) last week? What is the significance of a reactive NST?

5. What other test might she have ordered? Why?

6. What are the possible consequences of a pregnancy continuing past the established date (postdate)?

7. What is the most important nursing action after the rupture of the membranes?

8. Holly continued to eat lightly and drink fluids throughout her labor. Discuss the safety of this.

9. Describe the fetal heart pattern.

10. How are fetal heart tones (FHTs) monitored without an electronic fetal monitor at home?

11. Holly delivers a baby boy after 45 minutes of pushing in a squatting position over an intact perineum. The baby's APGARS are 9 and 10. She then immediately puts the baby to breast. Discuss the squatting position for pushing.

12. What is the advantage of not cutting an episiotomy?

13. The midwife does not cut the cord immediately, but places the baby on her mom and waits for the cord to stop pulsating. What are the advantages and disadvantages of this action?

14. Aside from the benefits of the quality of the breast milk, what is the particular advantage for Holly of breastfeeding?

References

Littleton, L., & Engebretson, J. C. (2002). *Maternal, neonatal, and women's health nursing.* Clifton Park, NY: Thomson Delmar Learning.

Jewell, Olsen O. (2004). Home versus hospital birth. *The Cochrane Library,* 3. Chichester, UK: John Wiley & Sons, Ltd.

Rabe, H., Reynolds, G., & Diaz-Rossello, J. (2004). Early versus delayed umbilical cord clamping in preterm infants. *Cochrane Database System Review, 18*(4): CD003248.

Varney, H., Kriebs, J., & Gegor, C. (2004). *Varney's midwifery* (4th ed.). Boston: Jones and Bartlett.

Leticia

AGE

15

SETTING

- Hospital urgent care center

CULTURAL CONSIDERATIONS

- Puerto Rican traditional beliefs

ETHNICITY

- Hispanic American

PRE-EXISTING CONDITION

- Obesity

CO-EXISTING CONDITION/CURRENT PROBLEM

- Precipitous delivery

COMMUNICATIONS

DISABILITY

SOCIOECONOMIC STATUS

SPIRITUAL/RELIGIOUS

PSYCHOSOCIAL

- Denial of pregnancy; no identified fob

LEGAL

- Minor

ETHICAL

PRIORITIZATION

- Immediate care of baby and mother after a precipitous birth

DELEGATION

PHARMACOLOGIC

ALTERNATIVE THERAPY

SIGNIFICANT HISTORY

- Primigravida

INTRAPARTUM

Level of difficulty: Easy

Overview: This case requires an understanding of adolescent behavior. It also requires critical thinking concerning legal implications regarding care of a pregnant minor.

Client Profile

Leticia is a 15-year-old, G1P0, SHF at 36-4/7 wga. She is visiting her sister in Florida (from Michigan) for a three-day weekend to get a break from the cold weather. Leticia is five feet two inches tall and weighs 168 pounds; she wears baggy clothes and is in complete denial of her pregnancy. Her parents, first-generation Puerto Rican immigrants (in Michigan), and sister are totally unaware that she is pregnant. Because of her denial, she has had no prenatal care.

Case Study

At 1 a.m. the night after her arrival in Florida, Leticia begins to get strong stomach "cramps." She does not tell her sister until they have gone on for most of the night. Finally, at 7 a.m. she wakes her sister in tears and tells her about "this awful stom-achache," she has. Her sister immediately decides to take her to the nearest urgent care center for treatment. Because she is only 15, she is admitted to the pediatric area of the center and immediately taken to an exam room because she is doubled over in pain. She has continued to wear her usual baggy sweat suit and has not yet faced up to the fact that she is pregnant. Five minutes after being put into the exam room the nurse enters to get her vital signs and take an assessment of her problem. The physician is just finishing suturing a small child's hand in the room next door. It takes the nurse about two minutes to realize what is happening. She barely has a chance to put on gloves to do an internal exam when Leticia begins to push hard and her membranes rupture. Within five minutes the nurse delivers a four-pound baby girl with APGARS of 9 and 10, who is screaming and pink. From examination the baby appears to be between 35 and 36 weeks gestation.

Questions

1. During a precipitous birth, what are the priorities for the baby?

2. What are the priorities for the mother?

3. Identify three OSHA concerns in this situation.

4. Is it possible for any woman to completely deny a pregnancy that goes nearly to term?

5. Is there any problem with Leticia receiving care as a minor without her parents present?

6. Who is the legal guardian of the baby?

7. What are the nursing priorities for the immediate postpartum?

8. How will the nurse prepare Leticia for her discharge with her baby?

9. Leticia still denies she ever had sex. How will the father be listed on the birth certificate?

10. Should the nurse suggest that Leticia breastfeed her baby?

References

Freda, M. (2002). *Perinatal patient education.* Philadelphia: Lippincott, Williams & Wilkins.

Rostant, D., et al. *Liability issues in perinatal nursing.* (1999). Philadelphia: Lippincott, Williams & Wilkins.

CASE STUDY 4

Lydia

EASY

AGE

23

SETTING

■ Private OB practice/hospital

CULTURAL CONSIDERATIONS

■ Traditional Colombian culture

ETHNICITY

■ Colombian

PRE-EXISTING CONDITION

■ Healthy female w/normal term pregnancy

CO-EXISTING CONDITION/CURRENT PROBLEM

COMMUNICATIONS

■ Non-English-speaking client

DISABILITY

SOCIOECONOMIC STATUS

■ Affluent

SPIRITUAL/RELIGIOUS

PSYCHOSOCIAL

LEGAL

ETHICAL

■ Cultural beliefs vs safety

PRIORITIZATION

DELEGATION

PHARMACOLOGIC

■ Epidural anesthesia

ALTERNATIVE THERAPY

SIGNIFICANT HISTORY

■ Primigravida

INTRAPARTUM

Level of difficulty: Easy

Overview: This case requires the learner to assess safety factors when they conflict with cultural practices.

Client Profile

Lydia is a 23-year-old, G1P0, MHF from Colombia visiting her sister in Miami, Florida. She does not speak English. She had only intended to visit her sister for a few weeks; however, political events in Colombia have made it impossible for her to return home. She has now been here two months and is 38 weeks gestation. She made an appointment at a private OB/CNM service to discuss her delivery. She did not bring her records since she never intended to be here this long. An initial OB visit is performed including all labs. Her sister is her interpreter. In Colombia, Lydia has already discussed with her obstetrician that she desires to have an elective cesarean section. She is from a prominent wealthy political family and considers vaginal delivery primitive and disgusting.

Case Study

Her initial prenatal visit reveals a healthy, 23-year-old, G1P0, MHF with a normally progressing intrauterine pregnancy (IUP) at 38 weeks gestational age. Her fundal height is 38 cm, there is positive fetal movement, the heart tones are in the LLQ in the 140s, all of her urine is negative, her VS are normal with a BP of 110/70, and she has no edema or headaches. Her personal and family history is benign. Her pelvis is gynecoid and adequate with blunt spines and pubic arch of over 90 degrees. Baby's estimated weight at this time is around six and a half pounds. As she is leaving, the nurse tells her that she needs to come back in one week. Her sister relays this to her and she seems upset. She tells her sister that she thought that she would be checking into the hospital for her cesarean section tonight.

Questions

1. What are the compared risks to the mother and the infant in a cesarean section versus vaginal delivery?

2. How should the nurse approach this situation?

3. Having a cesarean section is obviously a cultural norm for Lydia. At what point do respecting culture and the risk of compromising safe care begin to conflict? How do you prioritize this dilemma?

4. List at least three arguments that Lydia might use to justify her desire for a cesarean section. How should the nurse reply to each?

5. What are the possibilities that, if Lydia were to go into labor, she would still deliver by a cesarean section?

6. Are they increased over another woman who does not desire a cesarean section?

7. Lydia, against her wishes, is given an appointment to come back at 39 weeks. She tells her sister in Spanish, "This country is so backward. I would never have to tolerate this pregnancy this long back home." She then begins to cry. The sister explains this to the nurse. How should the nurse reply?

8. The nurse would like to offer Lydia some classes on labor preparation. How might this sensitive topic be approached?

9. At the 39-week visit, Lydia is obviously angry and again, through her sister, she insists on ending this pregnancy tonight with a cesarean section. "Why do they make me suffer so?" She asks her sister who interprets for the nurse. It is obvious that Lydia is used to getting her own way. Her BP is 148/76; FHTs at the left lower quadrant (LLQ) are in the 150s. She has lost two pounds in the past week and states that the baby is not moving as much as before. The obstetrician orders an NST that is reactive. Her Bishop score is 8. He also offers to induce her with an epidural if she wishes. Explain the BP elevation and weight loss. She accepts the induction if "I will not feel any pain."

10. What is a Bishop score?

11. Six hours into the labor with the epidural, Lydia has only dilated to 4 cm, is 100% effaced, and at zero station. She delivers via a cesarean section for failure to progress (FTP). Discuss this outcome.

References

ACOG News Release. (2003). Weighing the pros and cons of cesarean delivery. http://www.acog.org/from_home/publicatons/press_releases/nr07-31-03-3.cfm.

Blackburn, S. (2003). *Maternal, fetal, and neonatal physiology* (2nd ed.). St. Louis, MO: W. B. Saunders Co.

Cunningham, F. G., Gant, N., Leveno, K., Gilstrap, L., Hauth, J. C., & Wenstrom, K. (2001). *Williams Obstetrics* (21st ed.). Norwalk, CT: Appleton & Lange.

Howell, C. J. (2003). Epidural verses non-epidural analgesia for pain relief in labor. *The Cochrane Library,* 3. Oxford: Update Software.

Irion, O., & Boulvain, M. (2003). Induction of labour for suspected fetal macrosomia. *The Cochrane Library,* 3. Oxford: Update Software.

Levine, E. M., et al. (2001, March). Mode of delivery and risk of respiratory diseases in newborns. *Obstetrics & Gynecology, 97*(3), 439–442.

Peterson, G. (1981). *Birthing normally.* Berkeley, CA: Mindbody Press.

Rayburn, W. F., & Zhang, J. (2002). Rising rates of labor induction: present concerns and future strategies. *Obstetrics & Gynecology, 100*(1), 164–167.

Smith, G. C., Pell, J. P., & Dobbie, R. (2003). Caesarean section and risk of unexplained stillbirth in subsequent pregnancy. *Lancet. 362*(9398), 1779–1784.

Kathleen

AGE

21

SETTING

- Freestanding birth center

CULTURAL CONSIDERATIONS

ETHNICITY

- White American

PRE-EXISTING CONDITION

CO-EXISTING CONDITION/CURRENT PROBLEM

- R/o breech presentation

COMMUNICATIONS

- Deaf client

DISABILITY

- Deafness

SOCIOECONOMIC STATUS

SPIRITUAL/RELIGIOUS

- Christian Scientist

PSYCHOSOCIAL

LEGAL

ETHICAL

PRIORITIZATION

DELEGATION

PHARMACOLOGIC

ALTERNATIVE THERAPY

SIGNIFICANT HISTORY

- Multigravida

MODERATE

INTRAPARTUM

Level of difficulty: Moderate

Overview: Requires assessing a client for malpresentation and to rule out labor. Looks at communications with a deaf client.

Client Profile

Kathleen is a deaf, 21-year-old, G2P1001, MWF at 38 weeks gestational age. Kathleen has had a normal pregnancy throughout. She is very happy about the pregnancy and excited about the coming birth.

Case Study

Kathleen reports to the freestanding birth center at 1 a.m. with her husband, complaining of cramping for the past four hours and a vaginal discharge. Vital signs are: fetal heart tones (FHT) 140s, located just above and left of the umbilicus, with several accelerations heard while auscultating for two minutes, good fetal movement (FM); T 98°F, P 76, R 18, BP 110/68; contractions palpated every three minutes lasting 50 to 60 seconds and of moderate intensity with good resting tone. Her vaginal exam (VE) reveals 4 cm dilated and 80% effaced.

Questions

1. What questions does the nurse need to ask Kathleen to assess her contractions?

2. How do true labor contractions feel to the woman, as opposed to Braxton-Hicks contractions?

3. What is the significance of the FHT?

4. What further information is needed from the vaginal exam (VE) to assess her condition?

5. What is the significance of the vaginal discharge?

6. How will the nurse check to see if the membranes have ruptured?

7. If the baby were not engaged, would it pose a problem at this stage of labor?

8. What is the significance of the fact that she is deaf?

9. What is the best way for the nurse to communicate with Kathleen since she is deaf?

10. What is the significance if Kathleen's membranes are ruptured and meconium is present?

11. If Kathleen is in active labor, will she be allowed to deliver in the freestanding birth center?

References

Newbold II, H. (1979, March). Social work with the deaf: a model. *Social Work, 24*(2), 154.

Caissie, R. (2000). Conversation topic shifting and its effect on communication breakdowns for individuals with hearing loss. *Volta Review, 102*(2).

Herring, R., & Hock, I. (2000, February). Communicating with patients who have hearing loss. *NJ Medical, 97*(2), 45–49.

Iezzoni, L. I., O'Day, B. L., Killeen, M., & Harket, H. (2004, March). Communicating about health care: Observations from persons who are deaf or hard of hearing. *Ann Intern Med., 140*(5), 356–362.

Cassandra

AGE

24

SETTING

- Birth center to hospital transfer

CULTURAL CONSIDERATIONS

- Black-Muslim traditions

ETHNICITY

- Black American

PRE-EXISTING CONDITION

- Short stature

CO-EXISTING CONDITION/CURRENT PROBLEM

- Shoulder dystocia; GBS positive; FTP

COMMUNICATIONS

DISABILITY

SOCIOECONOMIC STATUS

SPIRITUAL/RELIGIOUS

PSYCHOSOCIAL

LEGAL

ETHICAL

PRIORITIZATION

DELEGATION

PHARMACOLOGIC

- Ampicillin; oxytocin (Pitocin)

ALTERNATIVE THERAPY

SIGNIFICANT HISTORY

- Multigravida

MODERATE

INTRAPARTUM

Level of difficulty: Moderate

Overview: Requires critical thinking to assess and identify treatment for shoulder dystocia.

Client Profile

Cassandra is a 24-year-old, G3P1011, MBF. She is five feet tall and her current weight at 40 weeks gestation is 142 pounds. Her pre-pregnant weight was 125 pounds. After 16 hours of active labor and being 6 cm, 100% effaced, and −2 station for six hours, she is transported from her planned home birth to the hospital. She is GBS positive and at the time of transport has already received two doses of ampicillin 1 gram each, six hours apart, by IV. Her membranes have been ruptured (SROM) for two hours. On admission to the labor unit her BP is 110/78, T 98.4, P 72, R 20. Contractions are q 5 to 6 minutes, lasting from 50 to 60 seconds, and strong at the peak (by palpation). The mother is having good relaxation between contractions. The FHT are reassuring with occasional accelerations: baseline of 130s to 140s and both long-term and short-term variability present. There are no decelerations. The estimated fetal weight (EFW) is 8 pounds. Her last baby was 7 pounds 10 ounces and was a normal spontaneous vaginal delivery (NSVD) at home with a licensed Muslim midwife. The baby is in a cephalic presentation left occiput anterior presentation (LOA). Reason for transfer: Maternal fatigue with failure to progress (FTP) in the last six hours with adequate contractions, which in the past three hours were becoming farther apart and weaker.

The obstetrician orders:

1. Pitocin IV to be increased every 20 minutes until contractions are coming every 2 to 3 minutes and lasting 90 seconds
2. Continue ampicillin 1 gram every 6 hours until delivery
3. Intrauterine pressure catheter (IUPC) and fetal scalp electrode (FSE) (Figure 2.2).

Case Study

Two hours following admission her contractions are every two minutes, strong, and 90 seconds in duration. Cassandra has requested an epidural anesthesia and is now resting.

The nurse notes the following at this time:

BP 100/60

Temperature 99

Pulse 82

Respirations 20

Vaginal exam (VE) 8 cm, 100%, −2 station

FHT 150s no accelerations, minimal variability, no decelerations, baby is moving during rest periods between contractions

Uterus is relaxed between contractions

A foley catheter has been inserted and output is sufficient

Figure 2.2 *Placement of an intrauterine pressure catheter and fetal scalp electrode.*

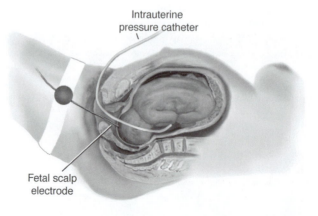

Intrauterine pressure catheter

Fetal scalp electrode

Questions

1. What is the significance of the baby still being at a negative 2 station?

2. Assess the following data: FHT 150s, no accelerations, minimal variability, no decelerations, baby is moving during rest periods between contractions.

3. What is the rationale for the ampicillin?

4. Cassandra had desired a natural home birth with no pain medications. What factors led up to her requesting an epidural?

5. Two hours later she is totally effaced and 10 cm dilated (complete, complete). With encouragement, she pushed for two hours and managed to push the head out. Immediately the head turtles. What does the term *turtle* mean?

6. What are the causes of shoulder dystocia (Figure 2.3)?

7. What position should the nurse assist Cassandra into in order to assist the obstetrician in the delivery of the shoulders? (List two possible positions that may be helpful at this time and explain why they can help.)

8. Distinguish between supra pubic pressure and fundal pressure (Figure 2.4).

9. Which one will help to deliver the shoulders and why?

10. What measures should the nurse take to prepare for immediate care of this newborn?

11. What possible injuries might this baby sustain as a result of this delivery?

12. What injuries might the mother sustain?

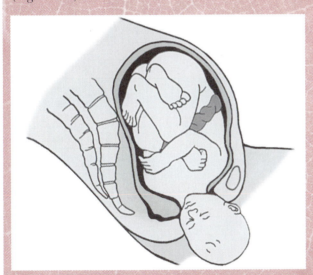

Figure 2.3 *Shoulder dystocia.*

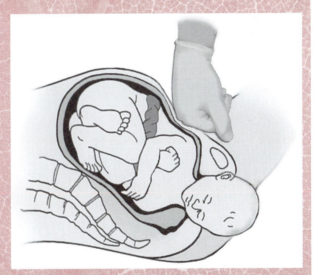

Figure 2.4 *Supra pubic pressure to release shoulder dystocia.*

References

Center for Disease Control and Prevention. http://www.cdc.gov.

Littleton, L., & Engebretson, J. C. (2002). *Maternal, neonatal, and women's health nursing.* Clifton Park, NY: Thomson Delmar Learning.

Varney, H., Kriebs, J., & Gegor, C. (2004). *Varney's midwifery* (4th ed.). Boston: Jones and Bartlett.

Mimi

AGE	**SPIRITUAL/RELIGIOUS**
36	■ Hindu
SETTING	**PSYCHOSOCIAL**
■ Hospital labor and delivery unit	
CULTURAL CONSIDERATIONS	**LEGAL**
ETHNICITY	**ETHICAL**
■ Indonesian American	
PRE-EXISTING CONDITION	**PRIORITIZATION**
CO-EXISTING CONDITION/CURRENT PROBLEM	**DELEGATION**
■ No prenatal care; moderate meconium staining	
COMMUNICATIONS	**PHARMACOLOGIC**
DISABILITY	**ALTERNATIVE THERAPY**
	SIGNIFICANT HISTORY
SOCIOECONOMIC STATUS	■ Multigravida

MODERATE

INTRAPARTUM

Level of difficulty: Moderate

Overview: This case requires using critical thinking to identify factors that interfere with normal fetal descent and identification of interventions to assist the infant to descend. It also requires identification of fetal heart tone patterns that indicate stress and abnormal contraction patterns.

Client Profile

Mimi is a 36-year-old, married, G3P2002, Indonesian female. This is her third pregnancy in three years. Like many Indonesian couples, she and her husband decided to put off having children until they had established their careers. She did not have prenatal care, and her due date is uncertain. Her fundal height is 36 cm. She is five feet six inches tall, and her current weight is 168 pounds.

Case Study

Mimi arrives at the hospital, with her sister and mother, in active labor. Her husband is with her but it is her mother and sister who assist her. She is admitted through the emergency room. She was 6 cm, 100% effaced; and the baby is at −1 station at the time of admission. Her membranes are ruptured, and the fluid is moderately meconium stained.

Questions

1. Shortly after Mimi is admitted to the labor suite she starts to push. The nurse checks her and finds that she is 7 cm and still at −1 station. What problems can result from Mimi's pushing at this time in the labor?

2. How can the nurse help Mimi stop pushing at this time?

3. What is the significance of the meconium in the fluid?

4. What special preparations will the nurse make to care for this infant immediately after birth?

5. The baby's head is in anterior asynclitism. What factors may account for this position?

6. The head engages. What problems can occur if the baby remains in a persistent asynclitic presentation?

7. What can be done to help direct the fetal head into the pelvis and convert the head to a synclitic presentation?

8. Three hours after admission the nurse notes that the baby's head is beginning to form a large caput. Fetal heart tones are noted to decrease to 110 bmp around the height of the contractions and return to the baseline of 130s just prior to the end of the contractions. What is the significance of these observations?

9. Bloody show is increasing and Mimi has an increased urge to push. The nurse checks her and finds that she has an anterior cervical lip. What might the nurse do to help reduce the lip and prepare Mimi to deliver?

10. After the lip is reduced, the baby begins to descend rapidly. The infant is crowning and the heart tones fall to 90s. The physician is preparing to deliver the head in the next few contractions. Identify two nursing actions that are appropriate at this time.

References

Cunningham, F. G., Gant, N., Leveno, K., Gilstrap, L., Hauth, J. C., & Wenstrom, K. (2001). *Williams Obstetrics* (21st ed.). Norwalk, CT: Appleton & Lange.

Nichols, F., & Humenick, S. (2000). *Childbirth education practice, research, and theory* (2nd ed.). Philadelphia: W. B. Saunders Co.

Vain, N. E., Szyld, E. G., Prudent, L. M., Wiswell, T. E., Aguilar, A. M., & Vivas, N. I. (2004). Oropharyngeal and nasopharyngeal suctioning of meconium-stained neonates before delivery of their shoulders: Multicentre, randomised controlled trial. *Lancet, 364*(9434), 597–602.

CASE STUDY 8

Danielle

AGE

41

SETTING

- Hospital labor and delivery unit

CULTURAL CONSIDERATIONS

ETHNICITY

- White American

PRE-EXISTING CONDITION

CO-EXISTING CONDITION/CURRENT PROBLEM

- AMA; older primigravida; augmentation; FTP; variable decelerations

COMMUNICATIONS

DISABILITY

SOCIOECONOMIC STATUS

SPIRITUAL/RELIGIOUS

PSYCHOSOCIAL

LEGAL

ETHICAL

PRIORITIZATION

DELEGATION

PHARMACOLOGIC

- Oxytocin (Pitocin)

ALTERNATIVE THERAPY

- Chinese medicine; Yongquan; Hoku; kidney 1; large intestine 4

SIGNIFICANT HISTORY

- Primigravida

MODERATE

INTRAPARTUM

Level of difficulty: Moderate

Overview: Requires assessing the pros and cons of induction and examination of the effects of interventions used to induce and augment labor.

63

Client Profile

Danielle is a 41-year-old, G1P0, MWF, who has experienced a normal pregnancy. She is five feet three inches tall and her current weight is 148 pounds. Danielle works as a bartender and due to the long hours on her feet she has experienced +2 pitting edema in both ankles. The swelling goes down when she lies down. Last week she told the nurse that she felt foolish because she had had a crazy dream where she thought she was giving birth to a litter of puppies. Afterwards she sighed and said, "I'm too old to be going through all of this."

Case Study

Danielle arrived at the hospital on Friday afternoon complaining of intermittent mild to moderate contractions for the past 12 hours. She denied ruptured membranes and bleeding. She is 39 weeks gestation. In the triage exam she was found to be 60% effaced, 1 cm dilatated, and −3 station. Her membranes were intact. Her contractions were 5 to 6 minutes apart, lasting one minute, and strong at the peak. The obstetrician decided to admit her to the labor and delivery suite and to artificially rupture her membranes (AROM) and begin Pitocin to augment her labor. Seven hours after her admission she was diagnosed with failure to progress (FTP). She had dilated to 2 cm and 100% effaced station −3 after six hours of Pitocin-augmented labor and an epidural. She was given internal fetal heart monitoring/internal uterine monitoring, which indicated a fetal heart rate baseline of 120 to 126 bpm with occasional accelerations for the first two hours. For the last hour of the labor she had a baseline of 140 to 142 bpm and an increasing number of variable decelerations. These decelerations stopped when she was placed on her right side. She was given a cesarean section. Her baby girl weighed 8 pounds and was 21 inches long. Her APGARS were 8 at one minute and 8 at five minutes with points taken off for tone and color.

Questions

1. Is there any significance to the fact that Danielle is 41 years old?

2. Is there any significance to the fact that this is her first pregnancy?

3. Discuss Danielle's dreams.

4. What is the significance of the +2 pitting edema in her ankles?

5. What are the advantages or disadvantages of cesarean section following labor as opposed to scheduled cesarean section?

6. List the indications and risk of artificial rupture of membranes (AROM).

7. Why do you think a cesarean section was done?

8. What is the difference between Pitocin induction and Pitocin augmentation?

9. Analyze the information given regarding the fetal heart tones.

10. Why did the variable decelerations stop after the client was positioned on her right side? What other positions might have been used?

11. What effect might having an epidural have had on this labor and the cesarean section outcome?

12. What else might have been done to help the baby descend and labor progress?

References

ACOG. Evaluation of cesarean delivery. (2000). Washington DC: ACOG.

American Academy of Pediatrics. (2005, February). Policy statement: Breastfeeding and the use of human milk. *Pediatrics 115*(2), 496–506.

Blackburn, S. (2003). *Maternal, fetal, and neonatal physiology* (2nd ed.). St. Louis, MO: W. B. Saunders Co.

CIMS Coalition for Improving Maternity Services. (2003). *The risks of cesarean section to mother and baby: a CIMS fact sheet.* http://www.motherfriendly.org/Downloads/csec-fact-sheet.pdf.

Fraser, W., Turcot, L., Krauss, I., & Brisson-Carrol, G. (2003). Amniotomy for shortening spontaneous labour. *The Cochrane Library,* 2. Oxford: Update Software.

Frye, A. (1995). Holistic midwifery care during pregnancy, 1. Portland, OR: Labrys Press.

Hodgess, S., & Goer, H. (2004). Effects of hospital economics on maternity care. *Citizens for Midwifery News.*

Howell, C. J. (2003). Epidural verses non-epidural analgesia for pain relief in labor. *The Cochrane Library,* 3. Oxford: Update Software.

Jacobsson, B., Ladfors, L., & Milsom, I. (2004, October). Advanced maternal age and adverse perinatal outcome. *Obstetrics & Gynecology, 104*(4), 727–733.

Levine, E. M., Ghai, V., Barton, J. J., & Strom, C.M. (2001). Mode of delivery and risk of respiratory diseases of newborns. *Obstetrics & Gynecology, 97*(3), 439–442.

Littleton, L., and Engebretson, J. C. (2002). *Maternal, neonatal, and women's health nursing,* Clifton Park, NY: Thomson Delmar Learning.

Lydon-Rochelle, M., Holt, V. L., Easterling, T. R., & Martin, D. P. (2001). First birth cesarean and placenta abruption or previa at second birth. *Obstetrics & Gynecology, 1:*97(5PT1), 765–769.

Scott, J. R. (2002). Putting elective cesarean into perspective. *Obstetrics & Gynecology, 99,* 967–968.

Waters, B., & Raisler, J. (2003). Ice massage for the reduction of labor pain. *Journal of Midwifery and Women's Health.* New York: Elsevier.

Young, A. (2002). Acupuncture pain relief for the midwife. *Acupuncture Newsletter,* Miami.

Josie

MODERATE

AGE	**SPIRITUAL/RELIGIOUS**
26	■ Episcopal
SETTING	**PSYCHOSOCIAL**
■ Birth center	
CULTURAL CONSIDERATIONS	**LEGAL**
■ American urban professional culture	
ETHNICITY	**ETHICAL**
■ White American	
PRE-EXISTING CONDITION	**PRIORITIZATION**
CO-EXISTING CONDITION/CURRENT PROBLEMS	**DELEGATION**
■ Prolapsed cord	
COMMUNICATIONS	**PHARMACOLOGIC**
DISABILITY	**ALTERNATIVE THERAPY**
SOCIOECONOMIC STATUS	**SIGNIFICANT HISTORY**
■ Professional	■ Multigravida

INTRAPARTUM

Level of difficulty: Moderate

Overview: This case requires identification of risk factors associated with a prolapsed cord. It also requires that the student identify the appropriate emergency care required when a prolapsed cord occurs.

Client Profile

Josie is a 26-year-old, G2P1001, MWF. Her pregnancy has been uneventful. She and her husband are very happy about this pregnancy. Their first child is three years old. Josie is a secondary school math teacher. She has remained employed throughout the pregnancy until last week when voiding frequency and urgency, and shortness of breath became such problems that she decided to take a leave until after the baby is born. They plan to deliver at the birth center where their first child was born. Josie's pregnancy is at 38 weeks gestation. She was just seen in the office this morning, and she and baby were doing well. The urine chemstrip was negative; BP and FHT were normal. The baby was at a −1 to −2 station, and her cervix was 80% effaced and 2 cm dilatated. Josie had lost two pounds since last week. She had no edema and no headaches or vision changes. At that time she was not experiencing any contractions.

Case Study

At 1 a.m. Josie and her husband call the midwife to tell her that Josie's waters have broken, and they are going to the birth center. When the midwife greets them Josie is smiling and relaxed. She has been having contractions for about four hours at home, and they are just beginning to get strong. The baby is active. Immediately upon getting to the birth center Josie asks to use the toilet. As soon as she sits down she tells the midwife that something is coming out of her vagina. The midwife recognizes a prolapsed cord (Figure 2.5).

Figure 2.5 *Prolapsed cord.*

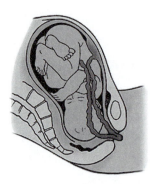

Questions

1. The midwife calls the nurse to assist in positioning Josie. What position will they place her in?

2. What are the risks associated with prolapsed cord?

3. What factors contributed to the cord prolapsing?

4. While the midwife does a vaginal exam, the nurse checks the fetal heart tones. What patterns might the nurse expect to hear?

5. What other immediate actions are needed at this time?

6. Should the cord be replaced into the vagina?

7. Josie is to be transported to the hospital. How should this transport be accomplished?

8. At the hospital Josie is given an emergency cesarean section. (It is less than 30 minutes since she first entered the birth center.) The baby's APGARS are 2 at one minute, 5 at five minutes, and then 6 at ten minutes. The baby is put on a ventilator and admitted to the neonatal intensive care unit. Within eight hours the baby is able to be removed from the ventilator and is doing well. What problems can be anticipated for this baby?

9. What problems might the mother experience postpartum?

References

Simpson, K. R., & Creehan, P. A. (2001). *AWHONN perinatal nursing* (2nd ed.). Philadelphia: Lippincott, Williams & Wilkins.
Varney, H., Kriebs, J., & Gegor, C. (2004). *Varney's midwifery* (4th ed.). Boston: Jones and Bartlett.

Jennifer

AGE

17

SETTING

- Hospital labor and delivery unit

CULTURAL CONSIDERATIONS

- Black American

ETHNICITY

- Black American

PRE-EXISTING CONDITION

CO-EXISTING CONDITION/CURRENT PROBLEM

- Preterm labor with spontaneous rupture of membranes (SROM)

COMMUNICATIONS

DISABILITY

SOCIOECONOMIC STATUS

- Low income

SPIRITUAL/RELIGIOUS

PSYCHOSOCIAL

LEGAL

- Minor

ETHICAL

PRIORITIZATION

DELEGATION

PHARMACOLOGIC

ALTERNATIVE THERAPY

- Transcutaneous electrical stimulation (TENS); sterile water papules

SIGNIFICANT HISTORY

- Primigravida

INTRAPARTUM

Level of difficulty: Difficult

Overview: This case requires that students be able to visualize the rotation of the fetus to identify problems with OP presentations. Students need to have knowledge of the role of the doula as well as knowledge of comfort measures. Furthermore, they must identify when labor stimulation is and is not appropriate. It requires them to determine how appropriate pain medication is in the later part of active labor, means of determining ROM, and assessment of labor progress.

DIFFICULT

Client Profile   **Jennifer** is a 17-year-old, G1P0, MBF. Jennifer is an active high school senior. She attended childbirth classes held at her high school. She attends a special program for pregnant teens. She has been careful to eat well and avoid all hazards that might harm her baby. She is looking forward to holding her baby and does not appear to be afraid of the coming labor.

Case Study   Jennifer is admitted in active labor at 36-2/7 weeks gestation. She has been experiencing contractions for the past six hours. For the past two hours they have been getting stronger and lasting up to one minute each. She believes that her membranes may have ruptured. She is accompanied by her husband, her mother, and a doula. Upon examination, the nurse determines that she is 3 cm dilatated; 90% effaced, and at a station of −3. The baby's heart tones are 120s with no decelerations. The nurse confirms that her membranes have ruptured spontaneously (SROM). According to Jennifer this occurred two hours ago. Contractions are one minute in length, q 5 minutes, strong with good relaxation between contractions.

Questions

1. What is the role of the doula?

2. How did the nurse determine if Jennifer's membranes have ruptured?

3. What is the significance of the findings from the pelvic exam?

4. What is the significance of the ruptured membranes in Jennifer's case?

5. What stage of labor is she in?

After six hours Jennifer is 5 cm, 100% effaced, and −3 station. The nurse notes that the baby is in an occiput posterior (OP) presentation. This presentation puts the hard back of the baby's head against the mother's spine. Descent is slower and more painful.

6. How does the baby's presentation impact the labor?

7. What comfort measures might the doula use to help Jennifer cope with the labor?

8. What positions might the mother use to help the baby rotate and descend?

Four hours later the mother is 8 cm, 100% effaced, and −2 station. The baby has rotated to the left occiput transverse (LOT) presentation. This turns the baby to face the mother's side and reduces the pressure on her back.

9. Jennifer complains that she needs to push. What are the consequences if she were to push at this point?

Jennifer does not progress in the next two hours, the baby is developing a large caput, and the FHT are now 150s with an occasional variable deceleration. Contractions are every two minutes, 90 seconds in length, and strong with good relaxation between. The obstetrician expresses concern that he may need to do a cesarean section. Jennifer asks for more time to see if she can begin to progress again.

10. Which of the following would be appropriate management of Jennifer at this point?

a. The doctor allows her two more hours to dilatate and orders Pitocin to make the contraction more effective.

b. She is given an epidural to help the baby rotate and descend.

c. She is given meperidine (Demerol) 50 mg for pain to help her relax.

d. Jennifer is given IV antibiotics.

e. The doula helps Jennifer assume a hands-and-knees position.

References

Blackburn, S. (2003). *Maternal, fetal, and neonatal physiology* (2nd ed.). St. Louis, MO: W. B. Saunders Co.

Eappen, S., & Robbins, D. (2002). Nonpharmacological means of pain relief for labor and delivery. *International Anesthesiology Clinician, 40*(4), 103–114.

Gentz, B. A. (2001). Alternative therapies for the management of pain in labor and delivery. *Clinical Obstetrical Gynecology, 44*(4), 704–732.

Hodnett, E. D., Gates, S., Hofmeyr, G. J., & Sakala, C. (2003). Continuous support for women during childbirth. *The Cochrane Library,* 3. Oxford: Updates Software.

Littleton, L., & Engebretson, J. C. (2002). *Maternal, neonatal, and women's health nursing.* Clifton Park, NY: Thomson Delmar Learning.

Nichols, F., & Humenick, S. (2000). *Childbirth education practice, research, and theory.* Philadelphia: W. B. Saunders Co.

Simkin, P. (2001). *The birth partner* (2nd ed.). Boston: The Harvard Common Press.

Multiple Clients

SETTING

- Hospital labor unit

CULTURAL CONSIDERATIONS

ETHNICITY

- Varied

PRE-EXISTING CONDITION

CO-EXISTING CONDITION/CURRENT PROBLEM

- Meconium stained fluid

COMMUNICATIONS

DISABILITY

SPIRITUAL/RELIGIOUS

PSYCHOSOCIAL

LEGAL

- Need for nursing supervisor to be notified of increased staffing needs and inability to contact MD

ETHICAL

PRIORITIZATION

- Delayed starting epidural anesthesia without ability to monitor client for potential complication

DELEGATION

- Responsibility that can be given to the labor room technician

PHARMACOLOGIC

- Epidural; oxytocin (Pitocin)

ALTERNATIVE THERAPY

INTRAPARTUM

Level of difficulty: Difficult

Overview: This case involves asking the student to look at staffing in a very busy labor unit and to prioritize care based on immediate need. Four laboring mothers are presented who are all in need of nursing care from two RNs and a technician. The student is expected to identify the need for going outside the unit to seek assistance from the nursing supervisor and placing a call to any OB in the house when the physician is delayed in transit to the hospital. The student is also expected to be assertive in not allowing interventions with potential adverse effects to be done until adequate nursing staff can be assigned.

DIFFICULT

Unit Profile

Mt. St. Vincent Hospital is a 300-bed general hospital. The maternity unit is a level I. There are four beds in the labor unit and an early labor lounge. It is 11:30 p.m., and the second shift just came on duty.

Case Study

There are three clients already admitted in labor. The first client admitted to the unit is Jeanette, a 26-year-old SWF, primigravida at 41 weeks gestation. She was admitted three hours ago at 100% effacement and 3 cm dilatated. The baby is at zero station. Her membranes are intact.

The second client in labor is Frances, a 39-year-old married Haitian American multigravida who was admitted yesterday morning with preterm, premature rupture of membranes at 36 weeks gestation. She is being induced with Pitocin and her last vaginal exam was done at 11:15 p.m. She had progressed to 6 cm, 100% effaced; and the baby is at +2 station. Her vital signs at 11:00 p.m. were temperature 100.2, pulse 88, respirations 24, and BP 130/88.

The third client is Ida, a 17-year-old SWF, primigravida who was admitted two hours ago after being in labor at home all day. Two hours ago a vaginal exam (VE) revealed that she was 6 cm, 100% effaced; and the baby was at +1 station. Her membranes broke earlier in the day at home.

Questions

1. There are two RNs and one labor technician on duty tonight. While change of shift report was being given the following requests from the women were received at the nurses' station. At 11:30 p.m.:

1. Frances is asking for an epidural.

2. Jeanette wants to take off the electronic fetal monitor and walk around.

3. Ida wants to get up and use the bathroom.

There is also a call from admitting that a new client has just arrived and needs to be brought to the labor unit. The labor unit is expected to send someone to transport her. The clerk at the admission desk said that she seems to be in very active labor. This is her fourth baby.

Which clients need the most immediate attention?

2. At 11:50 p.m. while walking around in her room, Jeanette's membranes rupture. The fluid is dark greenish with particles in it. It also has a foul odor. When the nurse checks the baby's heart rate she hears an increase in the fetal heart tones prior to a contraction, a sharp drop, and then a rapid return with the heart tones going above the baseline for a few seconds after the contraction. Describe the nursing actions that are appropriate at this time and give the rationales for each.

3. Ida complains that she needs to have a bowel movement. She is irritable and refuses to continue her breathing with her doula. Her legs are shaking and she feels nauseated and begins to vomit. The nurse knows that these are all signs of what?

4. The new client is Julie, a multigravida admitted to the labor unit at 12 midnight. She is found to be 100% effaced, 9 cm dilatated; and the baby is at +3 station. She tells the nurse that she feels the urge to push. She is also demanding pain medication. How should the nurse respond to this client?

5. At 12:05 a.m. Ida is checked by one of the RNs and found to be 10 cm dilatated, 100% effaced; and the baby is at +1 station. The fetal heart tones are 130s with accelerations and no decelerations. She says she is tired and does not feel like pushing. What nursing actions are needed at this time?

6. Describe the best use of the staffing at 12:10 a.m.

7. At 12:20 a.m. the technician notifies the RN that Jeanette's fetal heart tones have decreased to 90 bmp for the past one minute and have not returned to the baseline. The nurse has instructed the technician to turn her to her side and start her on oxygen. A call was placed to her doctor 20 minutes ago when her membranes ruptured and meconium was noted. The physician has not returned the call as yet. The fetal heart tones do not improve when she is placed on her side. What nursing actions are required at this time?

8. The nurse anesthetist arrives to do the epidural for Frances at 12:30 a.m. The anesthetist tells the nurse that she has to get back to surgery as soon as possible and wants to quickly get the epidural started. Prior to the epidural being given, what nursing care needs to be completed?

9. At 12:25 a.m. Jeanette's physican calls. He is on his way to the hospital but is caught in a traffic jam and will be there within 15 minutes. He tells the nurse to have Jeanette prepared for a cesarean section and then to notify the surgical area to prepare for her.

What nursing actions need to be done to prepare her for surgery?

10. Prior to the epidural being started Frances complains about the need to push. The nurse checks her and finds her to be only 8 cm dilatated. What would the consequences be if she started to push at this time?

References

Hofmeyr, G. J. (2004). Prophylactic intravenous preloading for regional analgesia in labour. *Cochrane Review.* http://www.medscape.com/viewarticle/485124?src=search.

Daniel-Spiegel, E., Weiner, Z., et al. (2004). For how long should oxytocin be continued during induction of labour? *BJOG: An International Journal of Obstetrics & Gynaecology, 111*(4), 331–334.

Margaret

AGE

22

SETTING

- Hospital labor and delivery unit

CULTURAL CONSIDERATIONS

- Accepts American medicalization concepts of pregnancy and birth

ETHNICITY

- Black American

PRE-EXISTING CONDITION

CO-EXISTING CONDITION/CURRENT PROGRAM

- Amniotic fluid embolism; placental abruption; disseminated intravascular coagulopathy (DIC)

COMMUNICATIONS

DISABILITY

SOCIOECONOMIC STATUS

- Lower middle class

SPIRITUAL/RELIGIOUS

PSYCHOSOCIAL

LEGAL

ETHICAL

PRIORITIZATION

- CPR; client needs in an emergency

DELEGATION

PHARMACOLOGIC

ALTERNATIVE THERAPY

SIGNIFICANT HISTORY

- Multigravida

DIFFICULT

INTRAPARTUM

Level of difficulty: Difficult

Overview: This case requires recognition of an amniotic fluid embolism with development of DIC during a normal labor, nursing assessment of client condition, and prioritizing nursing care in an emergency delivery.

Client Profile

Margaret is a 22-year-old, MBF who recently moved to Georgia from Detroit. She is a G3P2002 and currently at 38 wga. Margaret started prenatal care at 8 weeks gestation. She is five feet four inches tall and her current weight is 130 pounds. Her total weight gain thus far is 18 pounds. She works as a telemarketer 10 hours a day, 5 days a week. She eats fast foods but loves to snack on raw vegetables. Her last baby was born five years ago, full term, and without complications. She was not happy about the birth but endured it, and now is feeling apprehensive about this coming birth. She just wants it over with so that she can get on with her life. Her husband plans to stay with her in labor as does her mother and a sister. She has decided to get an epidural (she had one last time) as soon as the labor becomes "too much to handle."

Case Study

Margaret is being seen today at the prenatal clinic because of a complaint of decreased fetal movement. A biophysical profile reveals a healthy baby with good tone, movement, adequate amniotic fluid, breathing movements, and a reactive non-stress test. The baby is estimated to be approximately 7 pounds. Her first baby was 6 pounds 9 ounces. Her cervix is soft, anterior, 30% effaced, and 1 cm dilatated. She is experiencing occasional weak contractions throughout the visit. The physician gives her the option of going to the hospital now and being induced, or waiting to go into labor. She decides to wait until the afternoon and then, if no regular contractions start, she will come in for an induction. Four hours later her contractions have started naturally at home. They are coming every three minutes and lasting a full minute when she arrives at the hospital.

Although she had planned to get an epidural early, she is doing very well with the contractions and finds that with the support of the nurse and the Jacuzzi bath, which the nurse encourages her to use, she is getting enough relief that she is considering not getting the epidural. Her labor progresses quickly, and within six hours of being admitted to the hospital she is completely effaced and 9 cm dilatated. The baby is at zero station. Her membranes rupture spontaneously while she is walking back to her bed from the bathroom, and before the nurse can even check the fetal heart tones Margaret cries out, short of breath, and holds her upper abdomen. The nurse gets her back to bed immediately, puts on the call light, and checks her BP and the baby's heart tones. Within a minute her BP drops to 60/40, she becomes faint and then becomes semiconscious, and the fetal heart tone baseline drops to 90 with a prolonged late deceleration. The physician is in the unit and immediately responds. Margaret is rushed to the OR, where a cesarean section is performed and a 6 pound 2 ounce baby boy is delivered. Even with full resuscitative efforts, the APGAR scores are 1 at one minute, 1 at five minutes, and 3 at ten minutes.

Margaret goes into cardiac arrest and is revived. Five minutes after her uterus is sutured from the cesarean section, and her abdomen is being closed, she begins to bleed profusely from every orifice and puncture site. A decision is made to do a hysterectomy while trying to correct her bleeding problem. Margaret has four IVs infusing with blood and expanders under pressure. Once again she is stabilized. An air ambulance is called in, and she is transported by helicopter to the regional high-risk center. Despite the immediate responses from the very beginning by the nursing and medical team, Margaret has another cardiac arrest on board the helicopter and dies. Her baby is also transferred to the high-risk center, and two weeks later he too dies.

Questions

1. Identify three possible causes for her sudden change in condition.

2. Could this problem have been identified prior to the actual crisis?

3. Did Margaret's use of the Jacuzzi tub increase her risk for this complication?

4. What labor factors have been associated with amniotic fluid embolism?

5. List, in order, the immediate nursing actions to be taken when Margaret cried out and within the first three minutes that followed.

6. On autopsy the precipitating problem identified was an amniotic fluid embolism. The immediate response was sudden hypotension, followed by a placenta abruption leading to hemorrhage, shock, and then disseminated intravascular coagulopathy (DIC). Discuss this sequence of events.

7. How frequently do amniotic fluid embolisms occur?

8. What lab tests should the nurse anticipate that the physician will order immediately?

9. List the steps in the neonatal resuscitation.

10. Margaret was being transferred from a small community hospital to a tertiary care center. What is the difference between the levels of maternity care?

References

Bowden, K., Kessler, D., Pinette, M., & Wilson, D. (2003, October). Underwater birth: Missing the evidence or missing the point? *Pediatrics, 112,* 972–973.

Bowen, M., et al. (2002). *Nurses drug guide* (4th ed.). Springhouse, PA: Springhouse Publications.

Cunningham, F. G., Gant, N., Leveno, K., Gilstrap, L., Hauth, J. C., & Wenstrom, K. (2001). *Williams Obstetrics* (21st ed.). London: Appleton & Lange.

Geissbuhler, V., Eberhard, J. (2000). Waterbirths: a comparative study. *Fetal Diagnosis and Therapy, 15*(5), 291–300.

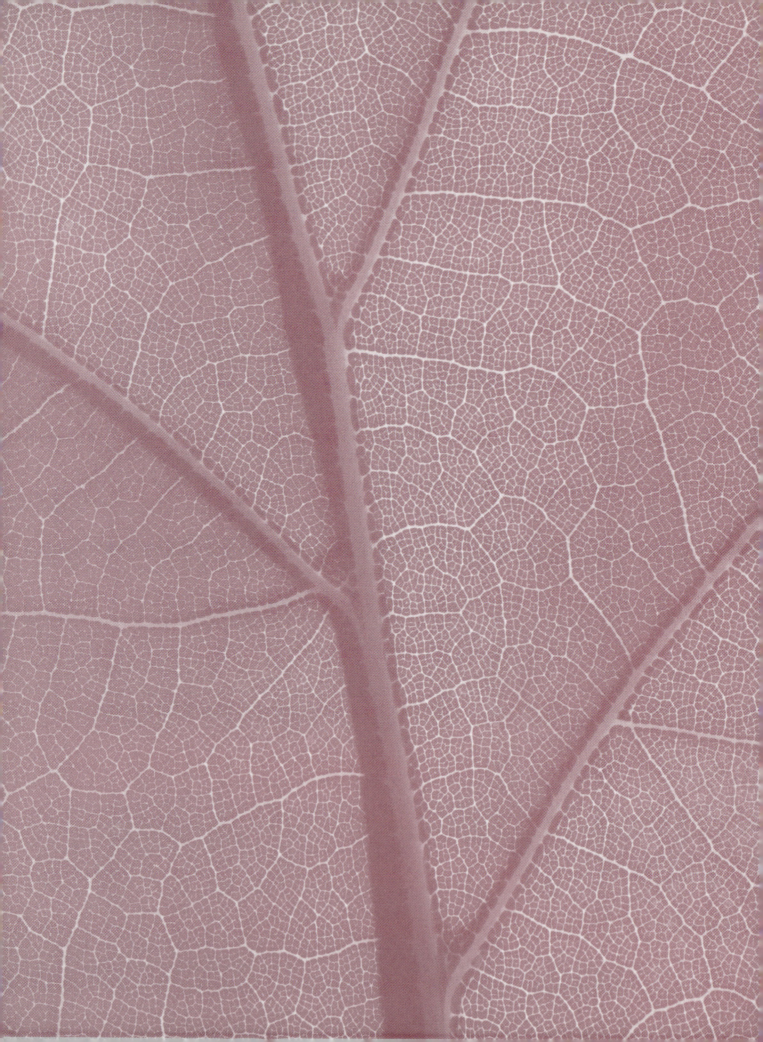

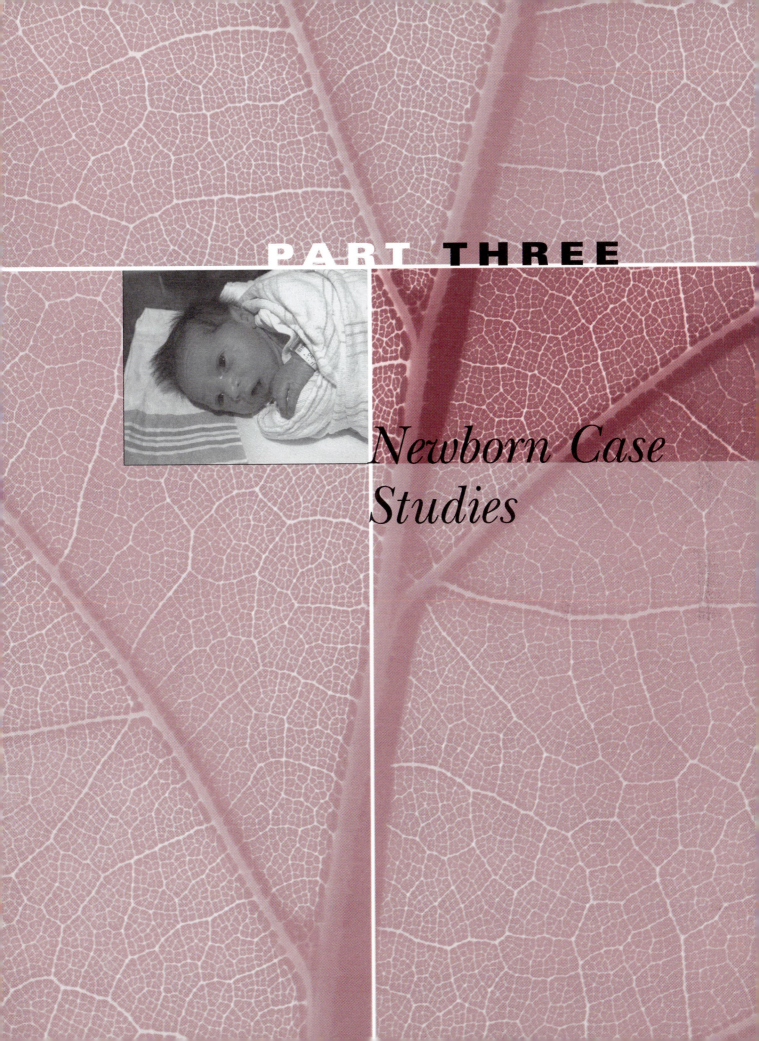

PART THREE

Newborn Case Studies

Baby Nova

AGE

24 hours

SETTING

- Hospital postpartum unit

CULTURAL CONSIDERATIONS

ETHNICITY

- White American

PRE-EXISTING CONDITION

CO-EXISTING CONDITION/CURRENT PROBLEM

- Initiating breastfeeding

COMMUNICATIONS

DISABILITY

SOCIOECONOMIC STATUS

SPIRITUAL/RELIGIOUS

PSYCHOSOCIAL

LEGAL

ETHICAL

PRIORITIZATION

DELEGATION

PHARMACOLOGIC

- Butorphanol tartrate (Stadol)

ALTERNATIVE THERAPY

SIGNIFICANT HISTORY

- Delivered by NSVD

NEWBORN

Level of difficulty: Easy

Overview: Requires that the student identify those factors that support and those that interfere with the initiation of breastfeeding. This case gives an example of a common hospital policy that can be detrimental to the mother/infant attachment process. It asks students to be cognizant of policies that may be outdated and are contrary to evidence-based studies. Furthermore, it asks students to consider the responsibility of the nurse in policy making and keeping care practices current with known research.

Client Profile

Baby Nova is 24 hours old. She is full term, weighs 7 pounds 3 ounces, and is 22 inches long. She was born via a NSVD after 12 hours of induced labor. Her mom had butorphanol tartrate (Stadol) for pain relief—last dose two hours prior to birth. After 10 minutes with mom and dad she was taken to the observation nursery until her temperature stabilized. Her APGAR scores were 8 and 9. Admission notes included T 98, HR 110, respirations 44, overall pink, active, and alert. She was given sterile water followed by 5% glucose by a bottle at two hours.

Case Study

The mother received Baby Nova at four hours of age and attempted to breastfeed for the first time. The baby had difficulty taking the nipple and after 30 minutes of trying, the mother, now in tears, called the nurse for help. Upon entering the room the nurse finds the mother in tears, and the baby is sleepy. She states, "She doesn't want the breast. Look, even when I can get her awake she just turns her head away from me." She is attempting to direct the baby's head toward the breast. The baby's maternal grandmother is with her. She is encouraging her daughter to give the baby a bottle since she perceives that her daughter does not have enough milk.

Questions

1. What is the rationale for taking the baby to the nursery for observation after the birth? As a nurse, how can you implement policy changes that reflect current evidence-based practice?

2. Why is Baby Nova given first sterile water and then 5% glucose feedings in the nursery?

3. Why do you think the baby will not feed when her mother offers her the breast?

4. What is happening when the baby looks away from the breast while the mother tries to direct her to the breast?

5. How does the pain medication given the mother affect her attempt to breastfeed at this time?

6. Describe proper positioning at the breast for breastfeeding.

7. Name three things that should have been done differently that would have increased this mother's ability to breastfeed this baby.

8. How can the nurse assist her now?

9. What are the consequences if the baby is given formula now?

10. The mother asks, "How long should I breastfeed?" What is the most appropriate answer?

References

American Academy of Pediatrics. (2005, February). Policy statement: Breastfeeding and the use of human milk. *Pediatrics, 115*(2), 496–506.

Anderson, G. C., Moore, E., Hepworth, J., & Bergman, N. (2003). Early skin-to-skin contact for mothers and their healthy newborn infants. *The Cochrane Library,* 3. Oxford: Update Software.

Biancuzzo, M. (2003). *Breastfeeding the newborn: Clinical strategies for nurses* (2nd ed.). St. Louis, MO: Mosby.

Crenshaw, J., et al. (2003). Case practices that support normal birth: No separation of the mother and baby after birth. *Lamaze International Education Council.* http://normalbirth.lamaze.org/institute/CarePractices/NoSeparation.asp.

Riordan, J., & Auerbach, K. (2005). *Breast feeding and human lactation* (3rd ed.). Sudbury, MA: Jones and Bartlett.

Uvnas-Moberg, K. (1998). Oxytocin may mediate the benefits of positive social interactions and emotions. *Psychoneuroendocrinology, 23*(8), 819–838.

Baby Haley

AGE

   Newborn

SETTING

   ■ Hospital delivery room

CULTURAL CONSIDERATIONS

ETHNICITY

   ■ Black American

PRE-EXISTING CONDITION

CO-EXISTING CONDITION/CURRENT PROBLEM

   ■ Down syndrome

COMMUNICATIONS

DISABILITY

SOCIOECONOMIC STATUS

SPIRITUAL/RELIGIOUS

PSYCHOSOCIAL

   ■ Grieving

LEGAL

ETHICAL

PRIORITIZATION

DELEGATION

PHARMACOLOGIC

ALTERNATIVE THERAPY

SIGNIFICANT HISTORY

   ■ Delivered by NSVD

NEWBORN

Level of difficulty: Easy

Overview: Requires recognition of signs of Down syndrome and critical thinking to assess and plan care for neonate with problems related to congenital anomalies.

Client Profile

Baby Haley's mother is a 26-year-old, G2P1001, MBF. Her first child is a healthy little 6-year-old girl. Mrs. Haley works as a cashier at Wal-Mart. There were no complications identified in the pregnancy, although she did not start prenatal care until her 24th week of pregnancy.

Case Study

Baby Haley has just been born after a two-hour second stage of labor. Immediately at delivery the nurse notes the following:

■ Baby Haley lacks tone. He feels like a "bean bag doll."
■ His color is dusky.
■ He made respiratory effort, but his breathing is irregular and shallow.
■ His heart rate is 100 bpm but irregular, with no murmurs.
■ When suctioned he reacted by sneezing and gagging.

After resuscitation the nurse continued to examine Baby Haley and further noted:

■ He had a large fat pad at the back of his neck.
■ He had simian creases on both hands.
■ His eyes seemed to be farther apart than usual.
■ His ears were low set.
■ His tone did not improve after resuscitation even though his color and respirations improved and he was weaned off the oxygen.

Questions

1. What is Baby's Haley's initial APGAR score? List the points for each component.

2. The mother was not screened for congenital anomalies. What might the reason be for this?

3. What congenital defects would the nurse suspect from the observed characteristics?

4. How diagnostic are these observations?

5. If the mother had started prenatal care earlier and had had a triple screen at 18 weeks gestation, what is the possibility that Down syndrome would have been identified?

6. If the triple screen or quad screen had come

back positive for Down syndrome, what further testing would have been reommended?

7. List the special observations that the nurse will make on Baby Haley during his transition.

8. The mother wants to nurse her son right after delivery. How should the nurse respond?

9. Baby Haley's mother asks the nurse, "What is wrong with him? My daughter seemed so different at birth." How should the nurse respond?

10. The father walks out of the delivery room, sits in a chair in the hall, and puts his head in his hands and cries. How should the nurse approach him?

References

Baliff, J. P., & Mooney, R. A. (2003, December). New developments in prenatal screening for Down syndrome. *American Journal of Clinical Pathology, 120,* S14–24.

Biancuzzo, M. (2003). *Breastfeeding the newborn: Clinical strategies for nurses* (2nd ed.). St. Louis, MO: Mosby.

Brigatti, K. W., & Malone, F. D. (2004, March). First-trimester screening for aneuploidy. *Obstetrical Gynecology Clinic of North America, 31*(1), 1–20.

Blackburn, S. (2003) *Maternal, fetal, and neonatal physiology* (2nd ed.). St. Louis, MO: W. B. Saunders Co.

Lawrence, R., & Lawrence, R. (1999). *Breastfeeding: a guide for the medical profession.* St. Louis, MO: Mosby.

Morris, K. (2004, April). *Prenatal screening for birth defects: an update. Missouri Medicine, 101*(2), 121–124.

Riordan, J., & Auerbach, K. (2005). *Breast feeding and human lactation* (3rd ed.). Sudbury, MA: Jones and Bartlett.

Tappero, E., & Honeyfield, M. E. (2003). *Physical assessment of the newborn* (3rd ed.). Petaluma, CA: NICU Ink.

Baby Maria

AGE

18 hours

SETTING

■ Postpartum unit

CULTURAL CONSIDERATIONS

■ Cuban American immigrant traditions

ETHNICITY

■ Cuban

PRE-EXISTING CONDITION

CO-EXISTING CONDITION/CURRENT PROBLEM

■ Milia; Mongolian spots; acrocyanosis; nipple confusion; formula supplementation

COMMUNICATIONS

DISABILITY

SOCIOECONOMIC STATUS

SPIRITUAL/RELIGIOUS

PSYCHOSOCIAL

■ Recent Cuban immigrant

LEGAL

ETHICAL

PRIORITIZATION

DELEGATION

PHARMACOLOGIC

■ Meperidine hydrochloride (Demerol)

ALTERNATIVE THERAPY

SIGNIFICANT HISTORY

■ Delivered by scheduled cesarean section

NEWBORN

Level of difficulty: Easy

Overview: This case requires that the student identify normal variations in the neonate. Requires identifying those problems created by cesarean section that interfere with breastfeeding and problem solving to reduce these problems.

Client Profile

Baby Maria was born via a repeat cesarean section at 38 weeks gestation in a large teaching hospital. Her mother is a 29-year-old G2P1001, recent Cuban immigrant.

Case Study

Baby Maria has been breastfeeding with formula supplement at night. Her mother is concerned about white spots on her baby's nose and chin and large "bruises" on her buttocks and upper legs. She is also concerned because the baby's feet seem cold and are bluish. Maria's mother asks the nurse to bring her some formula for the baby's afternoon feeding because she does not have enough milk and cannot find a comfortable position for nursing since she is in pain from the cesarean section.

Questions

1. How might the fact that Baby Maria was born by a cesarean section impact her mother's ability to be successful at breastfeeding?

2. What are the implications of Baby Maria being supplemented with formula at night?

3. How should the nurse respond to the mother's request for formula?

4. What suggestion might the nurse give to increase the mother's milk supply?

5. What positions might the nurse assist the mother in that will make her more comfortable for nursing after a cesarean section?

6. Explain the most probable cause of the "white spots on Maria's nose and chin"?

7. How should the nurse explain the "bruises" on the baby's buttocks and legs?

8. What explanation can the nurse give for the condition of the baby's feet?

9. Maria's mom is getting meperidine hydrochloride (Demerol) for pain relief. How can the nurse help Baby Maria's mother to relax and achieve the most effect from her pain medications?

References

American Academy of Pediatrics. (2005, February). Policy statement: Breastfeeding and the Use of Human Milk. *Pediatrics, 115*(2), 496–506.

American Academy of Pediatrics (AAP) and American College of Obstetricians and Gynecologists (ACOG). (2002). *Guidelines for perinatal care.* Elk Grove Village, IL: ACOG.

Freda, M. (2002). *Perinatal patient education.* Philadelphia: Lippincott, Williams & Wilkins.

Littleton, L., & Engebretson, J. C. (2002). *Maternal, neonatal, and women's health nursing.* Clifton Park, NY: Thomson Delmar Learning.

Baby James

AGE

6 hours

SETTING

- Small community hospital nursery

CULTURAL CONSIDERATIONS

ETHNICITY

- Black American

PRE-EXISTING CONDITION

- Fetal tachycardia

CO-EXISTING CONDITION/CURRENT PROBLEM

- Jaundice; low APGARS; hypoglycemia; hypothermia; coarse breath sounds; TTN; RDS

COMMUNICATIONS

DISABILITY

SOCIOECONOMIC STATUS

SPIRITUAL/RELIGIOUS

PSYCHOSOCIAL

LEGAL

ETHICAL

PRIORITIZATION

DELEGATION

PHARMACOLOGIC

ALTERNATIVE THERAPY

SIGNIFICANT HISTORY

- Delivered by NSVD at 36 weeks gestation; no prenatal care; prolonged ruptured membranes

NEWBORN

Level of difficulty: Moderate

Overview: This case requires that the student understand how stress increases the neonate's metabolic rate and the effects this has on the infant's ability to survive. Requires critical thinking regarding differentiating a benign respiratory problem (TTN) and the life threatening condition of RDS. Requires knowledge regarding developing jaundice in the neonate under 24 hours.

Client Profile

Baby James was born via a normal spontaneous vaginal delivery (NSVD) at 36 weeks gestation in a small community hospital. The mother arrived at the emergency room at 9 cm, 100% effaced, reporting ruptured membranes for 22 hours. Baby's fetal heart tones were 170 bpm. The mother delivered in the emergency room 30 minutes after being examined. This is her seventh pregnancy, and she did not have prenatal care.

Case Study

Baby James was admitted to the observation nursery from the emergency room where he was born. He weighed 5 pounds and was 19 inches long. His APGARS were 6 at one minute, and 8 at five minutes. Points were initially taken off for tone, reflexes, and color. His initial glucose was 35 and vital signs were HR 150, respiratory rate 76, temperature 97.2. The nurse noted some nasal flaring, grunting, and coarse breath sounds. He was given 1 ounce of D_5W PO, oxygen therapy; his skin and nasal pharynx were cultured, and he was observed on a warmer with skin probe for temperature monitoring.

At two hours the baby's glucose was 40, the nasal flaring continued, respiratory rate was 100 and irregular with continued coarse breath sounds. He exhibited acrocyanosis, and his temperature was 96.8. The baby was treated for transient tachypnea of the newborn (TTN) with oxygen therapy and a warm environment.

At four hours the nurse noted that the baby was lethargic and difficult to arouse. He appeared pale with circumoral cyanosis, nasal flaring, and grunting with sternal retractions. The nurse notified the pediatrician, an IV was started, and the baby was transferred to the neonatal intensive care unit (NICU) at a hospital in the next town.

At six hours the mother called the NICU to check on his progress and was told that he had subsequently developed jaundice and was on a ventilator.

Questions

1. What is the significance of the fact that this mother had no prenatal care?

2. What are the risks involved in a precipitous delivery?

3. What do you think might have been done differently for this delivery had the mother come in at 4 to 6 cm instead of 9 cm?

4. List the progressive signs of respiratory distress exhibited by this infant after birth.

5. This baby is initially being screened for infection and treated for transient tachypnea of the newborn. What data supports this diagnosis?

6. What is the most likely reason for this baby's initial hypoglycemia?

7. Assess the baby's vital signs. Which ones are within normal range and which ones need attention?

8. List the risk factors that existed for infection.

9. Why is this baby hypothermic, and how does it affect this baby's transition?

10. How significant is the acrocyanosis?

11. What is the significance of jaundice in a 6-hour-old infant?

References

Blackburn, S. (2003). *Maternal, fetal, and neonatal physiology* (2nd ed.). St. Louis, MO: W. B. Saunders Co.

Littleton, L., & Engebretson, J. C. (2002). *Maternal, neonatal, and women's health nursing.* Clifton Park, NY: Thomson Delmar Learning.

Simpson, K. R., & Creehan, P. A. (2001). *AWHONN perinatal nursing* (2nd ed.). Philadelphia: Lippincott, Williams & Wilkins.

Baby Ittybit

AGE	**SPIRITUAL/RELIGIOUS**
48 hours	
SETTING	**PSYCHOSOCIAL**
■ Home	■ Negative familial interference
CULTURAL CONSIDERATIONS	**LEGAL**
ETHNICITY	**ETHICAL**
■ Black American	
PRE-EXISTING CONDITION	**PRIORITIZATION**
CO-EXISTING CONDITION/CURRENT PROBLEM	**DELEGATION**
■ Physiologic jaundice	
COMMUNICATIONS	**PHARMACOLOGIC**
DISABILITY	**ALTERNATIVE THERAPY**
SOCIOECONOMIC STATUS	**SIGNIFICANT HISTORY**
	■ Delivered by NSVD

MODERATE

NEWBORN

Level of difficulty: Moderate

Overview: Requires using critical thinking to assess the neonate who is experiencing physiologic jaundice. This case also looks at factors that undermine a mother's confidence in breastfeeding.

Client Profile

Baby Ittybit is a 48-hour-old Black American neonate. He was born at the birth center two days ago. He is breastfeeding well and is active and alert.

Case Study

The nurse is making a home visit to check on the mother and baby. The maternal grandmother is very concerned about the baby since he appears yellow. She had discouraged her daughter from breastfeeding and wanted her to deliver in the hospital. She is convinced that the baby is getting sick due to breastfeeding and being born outside of an acute care facility. The mother is becoming very tearful and losing her confidence.

Questions

1. From an initial assessment, what is the main problem in this situation?

2. What is the most probable explanation for the baby being jaundiced? Give supporting evidence for your answer.

3. Explain the physiology of physiologic jaundice.

4. Baby Ittybit is Black American. How is jaundice assessed in darker skinned infants?

5. Explain how breast milk affects neonatal jaundice.

6. Is it probable that breast milk is the problem? Why or why not?

7. What observations can the nurse make that will help determine if the baby is experiencing pathologic jaundice?

8. List four causes of pathologic jaundice.

9. Describe the four steps of bilirubin metabolism.

10. What are the potential consequences if Baby Ittybit has pathologic jaundice and it is not treated?

11. Outline a teaching plan to educate the parents and grandmother about jaundice and to empower the mother on her ability to make decisions about her baby's care.

References

American Academy of Pediatrics. *Breastfeeding initiatives at the American Academy of Pediatrics.* http://www.aap.org/healthtopics/breastfeeding.cfm.

American Academy of Pediatrics. (2005, February). Policy statement: Breastfeeding and the use of human milk. *Pediatrics, 115*(2), 496–506.

Biancuzzo, M. (2003). *Breastfeeding the newborn* (2nd ed.). St. Louis, MO: Mosby.

Blackburn, S. (2003). *Maternal, fetal, and neonatal physiology* (2nd ed.). St Louis, MO: W. B. Saunders Co.

Littleton, L., & Engebretson, J. C. (2002). *Maternal, neonatal, and women's health nursing.* Clifton Park, NY: Thomson Delmar Learning.

Morrow Cavanaugh, B. (1999). *Nurses manual of laboratory and diagnostic tests* (3rd ed.). Philadelphia: F. A. Davis.

National Breastfeeding Awareness Campaign. (2004). http://4woman.gov.

Baby Chary

AGE

24 hours

SETTING

- Newborn nursery

CULTURAL CONSIDERATIONS

ETHNICITY

- White American

PRE-EXISTING CONDITION

CO-EXISTING CONDITION/CURRENT PROBLEM

- Potential hearing loss

COMMUNICATIONS

DISABILITY

SOCIOECONOMIC STATUS

SPIRITUAL/RELIGIOUS

PSYCHOSOCIAL

LEGAL

ETHICAL

PRIORITIZATION

DELEGATION

PHARMACOLOGIC

- Tetracycline; azithromycin (Zithromax); metronidazole (Flagyl); nicotine

ALTERNATIVE THERAPY

SIGNIFICANT HISTORY

- Delivered by NSVD

NEWBORN

Level of difficulty: Moderate

Overview: This case requires that the student understand the connection between maternal prenatal drug ingestion and neonatal hearing. The learner will also be asked to identify various integumentary alterations seen in the newborn.

Client Profile

Baby Chary was born 24 hours ago. Her mother went into labor at 38 weeks gestation and delivered after 16 hours of normal labor and delivery. The pregnancy was essentially normal with the exception that at the beginning of the pregnancy the mother was taking several medications prior to knowing that she was pregnant. The mother was taking a prescription of mocycline hydrochloride (Minocycline) and using topical erythromycin benzoyl peroxide (Benzamycin) gel for some facial acne. She was also taking birth control pills for several months during this period of time in which she was unaware of her pregnancy. The mother smoked a pack of cigarettes a day up to the time she discovered she was pregnant, but then used nicotine gum for a month while she reduced the number of cigarettes she smoked. Finally she was able to quit completely by four months gestation. During her second trimester she developed a severe sinus infection and was treated with prescribed azithromycin (Zithromax), 500 mg times one and then 250 mg a day for four more days. In the third trimester she was prescribed metronidazole (Flagyl) 500 mg bid for 7 days for a Trichomonas vaginitis infection.

Case Study

Baby Chary's APGARS at birth were 7 at one minute and 9 at five minutes, and the baby nursed well right after birth. The nurse notes the following features on an admission physical exam: preauricular skin tag on the right ear, a preauricular sinus on the left ear, and a large pink macular lesion on the back of the neck.

Questions

1. The mother stated that she never missed a birth control pill. What is the possibility of getting pregnant while not missing any pills?

2. What are the risks to the baby since the mother continued to take the birth control pills for the first two months of her pregnancy?

3. The mother asks the nurse what the pink mark is on her baby's neck. The nurse examines the mark and finds that it is small, approximately 1 cm flat with irregular edges. It blanches with pressure, and becomes darker as the baby cries. How should the nurse reply to the mother?

4. The mother notices that the baby does not seem to hear her. When and how will the baby's hearing be checked?

5. Review the medications that the mother took for the acne. What possible consequences do they present for the infant?

6. What is the significance of the skin tag on the baby's right ear?

7. On day three the pediatrician decided to look at the baby's ear canal with an otoscope. Describe how this procedure is done.

8. What are the advantages to early detection of hearing loss?

9. Discuss the mother's illness in the second trimester and her taking the azithromycin (Zithromax) at that time.

10. How does Trichomonas vaginitis affect pregnancy? How safe is metronidazole (Flagyll) in the third trimester?

11. Discuss the mother's use of tobacco and nicotine. Is Baby Chary at increased risk for any health problems because of it?

References

Blackburn, S. (2003). *Maternal, fetal, and neonatal physiology* (2nd ed.). St Louis, MO: W. B. Saunders Co.

Li, De-Kun, Daling, J. R., Mueller, B. A., Hickok, D. E., Fantel, A. G., & Weiss, N.S. (1995). Oral contraceptive use after conception in relation to the risk of congenital urinary tract anomalies. *Teratology, 51,* 30–36.

Simpson, K. R., & Creehan, P. A. (2001). *AWHONN perinatal nursing* (2nd ed.). Philadelphia: Lippincott, Williams & Wilkins.

CASE STUDY 7

Baby Cunningham

AGE

3 hours

SETTING

- Hospital

CULTURAL CONSIDERATIONS

ETHNICITY

- White American

PRE-EXISTING CONDITION

- Failed induction

CO-EXISTING CONDITION/CURRENT PROBLEM

- Prematurity; respiratory distress syndrome

COMMUNICATIONS

DISABILITY

SOCIOECONOMIC STATUS

SPIRITUAL/RELIGIOUS

PSYCHOSOCIAL

LEGAL

ETHICAL

PRIORITIZATION

DELEGATION

PHARMACOLOGIC

- Dinoprostone (Cervidil); oxytocin (Pitocin)

ALTERNATIVE THERAPY

SIGNIFICANT HISTORY

- Delivered by cesarean section following labor

NEWBORN

Level of difficulty: Difficult

Overview: Requires critical thinking in order to do gestational age assessment and identify respiratory distress syndrome. Requires identification of the effects of stress on temperature regulation, glucose stores, and respiratory transition.

DIFFICULT

Client Profile

Baby Cunningham was born three hours ago via a cesarean section for a failed induction following a normal pregnancy. The mother had come to the hospital with her membranes intact and having some moderate intermittent Braxton Hicks uterine contractions for the past 24 hours. A vaginal exam revealed a long and thick cervix, which was somewhat anterior and closed. The baby's gestational age was established at 37 weeks by late ultrasound because of an uncertain LMP. Since she was near term and her exam revealed that she was not in active labor, the decision was made to try to induce labor. She was started with a prostaglandin agent dinoprostone (Cervidil), for cervical ripening, then IV oxytocin (Pitocin) to induce and augment labor. She was given an epidural just after the Pitocin was started. Contractions were established at 90 seconds, coming every two minutes. After more than eight hours of labor, her cervix had effaced 60% and only dilated to about 1 cm. The baby developed some repeated prolonged deep late decelerations with poor recovery and minimal short-term variability. Because of the fetal distress, it was decided to turn off the oxytocin (Pitocin) and perform an emergency cesarean section for fetal distress and failure to progress. At delivery the infant was very pale with an extremely slow heart rate, no respiratory effort, and absent tone. Resuscitation included positive pressure ventilation (PPV) by bag and mask with short-term CPR. The baby's APGARS were 3 at one minute, 6 at five minutes, and 8 by ten minutes without any need for epinephrine or sodium bicarbonate. At birth the nurse noticed the following physical characteristics:

■ Large amount of lanugo and vernix
■ Breasts flat without buds
■ Faint plantar creases only
■ Equally prominent clitoris and minora
■ Slow recoil of ears

The neuromotor exam was not performed due to the persistent depression of the infant's tone and reflexes status post-resuscitation.

Case Study

Baby Cunningham was shown to her parents and transferred to the special care nursery for observation and continued support including oxygen and oxygen saturation monitoring. Under the radiant warmer (Figure 3.1), at 30 minutes of life, the baby was pale and breathing at 88 b/m with some nasal flaring and audible grunting present with some rales heard bilaterally with a stethoscope. Baby Cunningham was continued on blow-by oxygen, warmth, and suctioning prn.

At 45 minutes the respirations were still 88 to 100, with audible grunting, sternal retractions, and nasal flaring. The baby was pale, cyanotic, and dusky even on 100% oxygen by oxyhood with a pulseox saturation of 87%. Her heart rate was 190, and the temperature continued low at 96 in spite of active warming. Random blood glucose was 25 at one hour. The physician ordered an IV to be started with 10% glucose and blood cultures to be done.

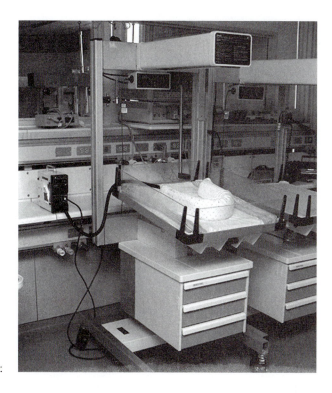

Figure 3.1 *Radiant warmer.*

Questions

1. What is the most likely cause of this infant's distress?

2. List the dangers of elective induction.

3. How accurate are late ultrasounds for establishing gestational age?

4. What is the normal respiratory rate of a neonate at this age? How does Baby Cunningham's compare? Why do you think this is occurring?

5. Assess Baby Cunningham's temperature. Is this normal at this age? Why do you think this is occurring?

6. What is the normal range for neonatal glucose levels? How does Baby Cunningham's compare? Why do you think this is happening, and what problems could arise if it is not corrected?

7. Explain the compensatory principles behind tachypnea, nasal flaring, grunting, and retractions in respiratory distress.

8. How does the environmental temperature affect Baby Cunningham's chances of survival?

9. Why were cultures done?

10. How does the APGAR score differ for the preterm infant as opposed to the full-term one?

11. How might this situation have been avoided?

12. What affects related to parenting can be expected as a result of the birth complications and infant condition?

13. How can the nurse minimize these consequences?

References

Blackburn, S. (2003). *Maternal, fetal, and neonatal physiology* (2nd ed.). St. Louis, MO: W. B. Saunders Co.

Kramer, M. S, Demissie, K., Platt, R. W., Sauve, R., & Liston, R. (2000). The contribution of mild and moderate preterm birth to infant mortality. *JAMA, 284*(7), 843–849.

Littleton, L., & Engebretson, J. C. (2002). *Maternal, neonatal, and women's health nursing.* Clifton Park, NY: Thomson Delmar Learning.

Rayburn, W. F., & Zhang, J. (2002). Rising rates of labor induction: present concerns and future strategies. *Obstetrics & Gynecology, 100*(1), 164–167.

Baby Long

AGE

   2 hours

SETTING

   ■ Hospital NB nursery

CULTURAL CONSIDERATIONS

ETHNICITY

   ■ White American

PRE-EXISTING CONDITION

CO-EXISTING CONDITION/CURRENT PROBLEM

   ■ Thrombocytopenia

COMMUNICATIONS

DISABILITY

SOCIOECONOMIC STATUS

SPIRITUAL/RELIGIOUS

PSYCHOSOCIAL

LEGAL

ETHICAL

PRIORITIZATION

DELEGATION

PHARMACOLOGIC

ALTERNATIVE THERAPY

SIGNIFICANT HISTORY

   ■ Cesarean section

DIFFICULT

NEWBORN

Level of difficulty: Difficult

Overview: The case examines the relationship of placenta abruption and development of thrombo-cytopenia in the newborn. The learner is asked to identify risk factors for and signs and symptoms in the neonate, identify risks associated with thrombocytopenia, and plan the care for the infant.

Client Profile   **Baby Long** was delivered by an emergency cesarean section two hours ago because of some fetal tachycardia and maternal fever of 101.8. The pregnancy was complicated by preterm premature rupture of membranes (PPROM), which occurred following an automobile accident two days ago at which time the mother sustained some minor trauma to the abdomen. During the delivery it was noted that she had developed a small to moderate placenta abruption. The baby's gestational age was determined to be about 32 weeks. The mother later developed disseminated intravascular coagulopathy (DIC) and is currently in critical condition in the Intensive Care Unit.

Case Study   The baby required full resuscitation at birth and had APGARS of 4 and 5 at one and five minutes. The ten minute APGAR was 6. She was immediately admitted to the NICU on a ventilator.

Questions

1. During the initial exam the nurse notes that the baby had petechiae on his abdomen and face and also notes that there is some oozing of blood from the venipuncture sites. List possible causes of this finding.

2. The nurse puts a call in to the physician. What initial laboratory studies should the nurse anticipate?

3. How might results be affected if the nurse decides to collect the blood for these tests by a heel stick?

4. The baby's platelet count is 60,000 units per liter. Assess this finding.

5. What would be the next anticipated set of lab tests that might be needed?

6. Would the nurse anticipate a spinal tap to be a part of the sepsis workup?

7. Should the nurse anticipate the insertion of an umbilical arterial catheter?

8. What other signs might the nurse note that would be associated with thrombocytopenia?

9. Baby Long was also diagnosed with intraventricular hemorrhage (IVH). What factors contributed directly to this condition?

10. List all of possible etiologies that are present in the delivery history.

11. What further lab tests might be included in the evaluation of this thrombocytopenia?

12. What is the treatment that the nurse should anticipate for this infant's thrombocytopenia?

References

Bianchi, D. W., Crombleholme, T. M., & D'Alton, M. E. (2000). *Fetology: Diagnosis and management of the fetal patient.* New York; McGraw Hill.

Blackburn, S. (2003). *Maternal, fetal, and neonatal physiology.* Philadelphia: W. B. Saunders Co.

Creasy, R. K., & Resnik, R. (1999). *Maternal fetal medicine* (4th ed.). Philadelphia: W. B., Saunders Co.

Mercer, J. S., McGrath, M. M., Hensman, A., Silver, H., & Oh, W. (2003, September). Immediate and delayed cord clamping in infants born between 24 and 32 weeks: A pilot randomized controlled trial. *Journal of Perinatalogy, 23*(6), 466.

Taeusch, H. W., & Ballard, R. A. (2004). *Avery's diseases of the newborn,* (8th ed.). Philadelphia: W. B. Saunders

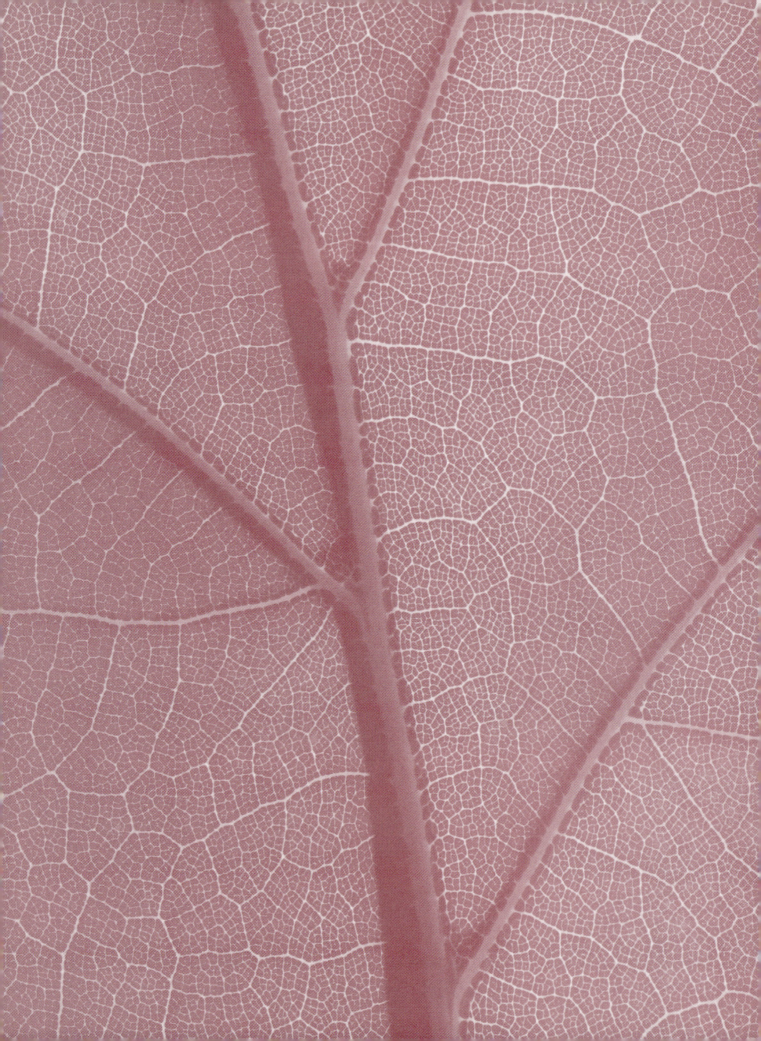

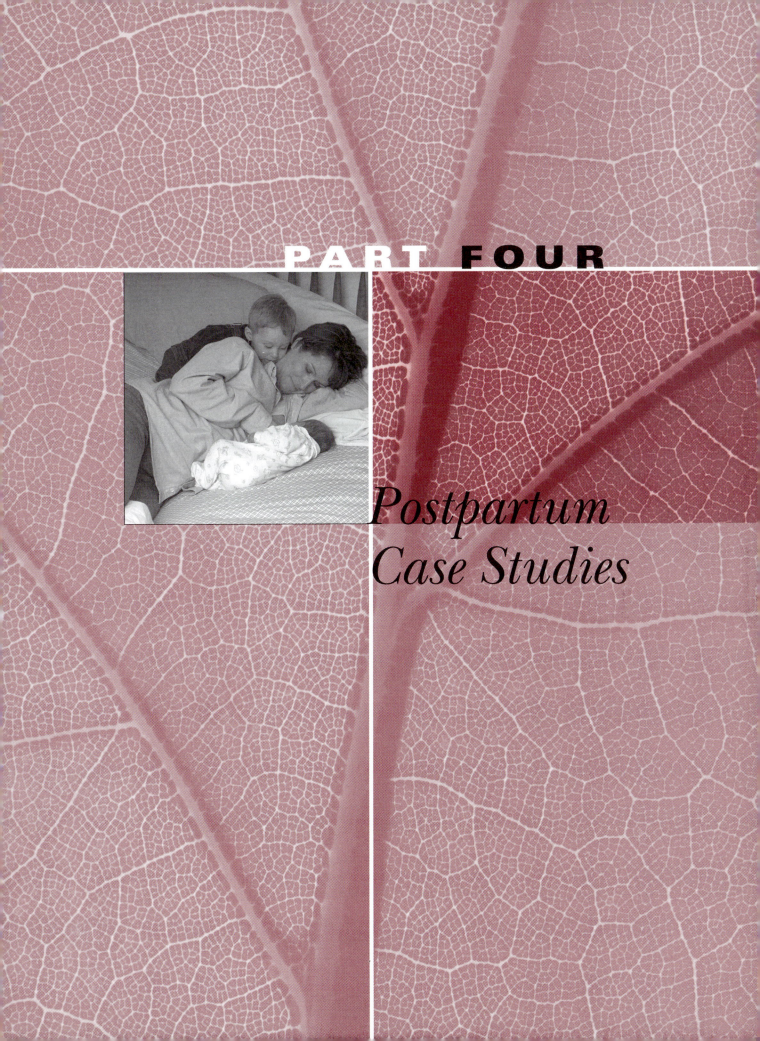

PART FOUR

*Postpartum
Case Studies*

Molly

AGE

29

SETTING

- Hospital postpartum unit

CULTURAL CONSIDERATIONS

- White American culture

ETHNICITY

- White American

PRE-EXISTING CONDITION

CO-EXISTING CONDITION/CURRENT PROBLEM

- PP blues; 4th-degree laceration; postpartum hemorrhage

COMMUNICATIONS

DISABILITY

SOCIOECONOMIC STATUS

SPIRITUAL/RELIGIOUS

PSYCHOSOCIAL

- Previous positive home birth experience

LEGAL

ETHICAL

PRIORITIZATION

DELEGATION

PHARMACOLOGIC

ALTERNATIVE THERAPY

SIGNIFICANT HISTORY

- Multipara

POSTPARTUM

Level of difficulty: Easy

Overview: Requires using critical thinking to assess and plan care for a woman experiencing postpartum blues following a postpartum hemorrhage and a fourth-degree laceration.

Client Profile

Molly is a 29-year-old, G2P2002, MWF. She is breastfeeding. Her first baby is two years old, and she breastfed that baby for one year. Her first baby weighed 8 pounds and was born at home, and she felt that it had been a wonderful experience. She delivered in the squatting position over an intact perineum, walked and danced throughout her labor, and used her bath to relax through much of the first stage. She had recently moved and could not find a midwife to help her with a home birth this time.

This delivery was induced at 40 weeks 2 days with Pitocin. After 6 hours she had an epidural for anesthesia. The baby was born vaginally with forceps. The baby weighed 7 pounds 2 ounces. She experienced a fourth-degree laceration following a mediolateral episiotomy. Her estimated blood loss (EBL) was 1000 mL.

Case Study

At 24 hours postpartum, Molly is feeling depressed. The nurse finds her crying quietly while breastfeeding her baby. The baby is feeding well. Molly's older baby is tucked in the bed next to her, asleep.

Questions

1. Make a list of possible reasons for Molly's tears.

2. What is the relationship between episiotomy and third- and fourth-degree lacerations?

3. What are the rationales for induction?

4. Molly had already experienced a natural birth and was satisfied with her birth. What factors may have caused her to ask for an epidural this time?

5. What pelvic structures are involved in a fourth-degree laceration?

6. What special precautions are needed for the woman who has a fourth-degree laceration?

7. What is the normal amount of blood loss for a vaginal birth?

8. How does Molly's loss compare?

9. List at least two complications that may occur as a result of her postpartum hemorrhage.

10. How should the nurse best approach Molly at this time?

11. If Molly's older baby wishes to resume breastfeeding, what should she do?

References

Himenick, S. (2003, March). Post ecstatic birth syndrome. *Vital Signs.*

Littleton, L., & Engebretson, J. C. (2002). *Maternal, neonatal, and women's health nursing.* Clifton Park, NY: Thomson Delmar Learning.

Simpson, K. R., & Creehan, P. A. (2001). *AWHONN perinatal nursing* (2nd ed.). Philadelphia: Lippincott, Williams & Wilkins.

Cunningham, F. G., Gant, N., Leveno, K., Gilstrap, L., Hauth, J., & Wendstrom, K. (2001). *Williams Obstetrics* (21st ed.). Norwalk, CT: Appleton & Lange.

Candace

AGE

23

SETTING

- Home

CULTURAL CONSIDERATIONS

ETHNICITY

- White American

PRE-EXISTING CONDITION

CO-EXISTING CONDITION/CURRENT PROBLEM

- Blocked duct; mastitis; postpartum blues

COMMUNICATIONS

DISABILITY

SOCIOECONOMIC STATUS

SPIRITUAL/RELIGIOUS

PSYCHOSOCIAL

LEGAL

ETHICAL

PRIORITIZATION

DELEGATION

PHARMACOLOGIC

- Ampicillin

ALTERNATIVE THERAPY

SIGNIFICANT HISTORY

- Primipara

POSTPARTUM

Level of difficulty: Easy

Overview: Requires using critical thinking to assess and provide care for a woman with mastitis.

Client Profile

Candace is a 23-year-old, G1P1, MWF who delivered a 7 pound 8 ounce baby boy three weeks ago at the local birth center. She is very happy about her birth and is adjusting well to motherhood. She breastfed her baby a few minutes after the birth and has continued to exclusively breastfeed him. She intends to breastfeed for at least a year, probably starting him on solid foods around six months. Prior to the pregnancy Candace was a busy office executive in a local shipping firm. She is on a six-week leave of absence. She plans to pump her breast milk for the baby when she returns to work. She is hoping that her mother-in-law, who will be caring for the baby, will be able to bring the baby to her workplace at least once a day, at noon, to breastfeed and then give the baby the breast milk she has left from a bottle for the other feedings. Her mother-in-law will be arriving from out of state in two weeks. Candace is a very "in control person." She plans everything in her life, and up to this point the world has respected her wishes.

Case Study

Candace called the birth center this morning crying. Her breast on the left side is so sore she cannot stand to have the baby nurse on that side, and to make matters worse, that is the only side the baby will take. For the last 12 hours the baby seems to want to nurse all the time or just cries and sucks his fist. She feels sick, cannot get anything done at home, and at 2 p.m. is still in her pajamas with last night's dinner and this morning's breakfast dishes still in the sink. She and her husband had an argument this morning and he left for work angry and overtired after getting no sleep all night from the baby crying. He just wants her to stop being so stubborn, since she obviously doesn't have enough milk, and give the baby some formula. Her car has broken down and she has no other source of transportation. The nurse working at the birth center offers to make a home visit.

Questions

1. Prior to arriving at the home, what problems does the nurse anticipate at this visit?

2. Make a list of the questions that the nurse will ask Candace at the home visit.

3. Make a list of the observations that need to be made at the home visit.

4. Explain the process of supply and demand as it applies to breastfeeding and milk supply.

5. Why does it appear to Candace's husband that Candace has lost her milk?

6. On arrival the nurse finds that Candace's left breast nipple is cracked and bleeding slightly. The nurse also notes that Candace has a fever of 101.2°, seems lethargic, and has an area about the size of a quarter on the underside of her right breast that is firm, red, and warm. Candace tells the nurse that she feels like she has the flu. What is Candace's problem, what probably caused it, and what is the nurse's next action?

7. The CNM at the birth center calls in a prescription for ampicillin 500 mg po qid for 10 days. Candace starts crying and asks if this means she can no longer breastfeed. What is the nurse's best response?

8. Outline a teaching plan to reduce the possibility of Candace having another mastitis infection.

9. Why did the baby only want to nurse on the left side?

10. How can the nurse help Candace get him to also nurse on the right side?

11. Where can the nurse refer Candace for support with her breastfeeding?

12. Candace plans to return to work in two weeks. Make a list of decisions and possible problems that she will have to work through during these next two weeks, and after she returns to work, to prepare her and the baby for this transition. Provide alternative suggestions for her to consider.

References

Biancuzzo, M. (2003). *Breastfeeding the newborn: Clinical strategies for nurses* (2nd ed.). St Louis, MO: Mosby.

Facts for Life: A Communication Challenge, produced for UNICEF, WHO, UNESCO, and UNFPA, rev. ed. 2002.

La Leche League International. (2003). *Leader's Handbook* (4th ed.). Schaumburg, IL: La Leche League International.

Littleton, L., & Engebretson, J. C. (2002). *Maternal, neonatal, and women's health nursing.* Clifton Park, NY: Thomson Delmar Learning.

Riordan, J., & Auerbach, K. (2005). *Breast feeding and human lactation* (3rd ed.). Sudbury, MA: Jones and Bartlett.

Juanita

AGE

24

SETTING

■ Home

CULTURAL CONSIDERATIONS

■ Cuban traditions

ETHNICITY

■ Cuban American

PRE-EXISTING CONDITION

CO-EXISTING CONDITION/CURRENT PROBLEM

■ Rh negative

COMMUNICATIONS

DISABILITY

SOCIOECONOMIC STATUS

SPIRITUAL/RELIGIOUS

PSYCHOSOCIAL

■ Cultural conflicts

LEGAL

ETHICAL

PRIORITIZATION

DELEGATION

PHARMACOLOGIC

■ Rh_o(D) immune globulin (human) (RhoGAM)

ALTERNATIVE THERAPY

SIGNIFICANT HISTORY

■ Primipara

POSTPARTUM

Level of difficulty: Easy

Overview: This case looks at some beliefs common in the Cuban culture, problems that arise from culture conflict between a mother-in-law and the husband, and differences between the daughter and her mother on expectations for postpartum. It also looks at the effects of emotional stress on the breast-feeding process.

Client Profile

Juanita is a 24-year-old, MHF. She is a gravida 1 para 1. Juanita emigrated from Cuba to Miami, Florida several years ago. She has a college education and has read everything she can get her hands on about pregnancy, infant care, and breastfeeding. Her mother just arrived from Cuba two days ago to stay with Juanita and her husband and to help care for her new grandchild. Juanita gave birth three days ago at the local community hospital. She and her husband are very happy about their new daughter. Juanita was discharged from the hospital with the baby yesterday. This morning she called the hospital saying that she was experiencing terrible constipation and was having problems breastfeeding. She asked for a nurse to come to her home for a home visit to help her.

Case Study

When the nurse arrives Juanita is alone with the baby. Her husband went grocery shopping and her mother has gone to the Laundromat^SM to do the washing. Juanita seems happy to see the nurse. They talk for a while and then Juanita bursts into tears. She explains to the nurse that her mother and her husband have been at odds since she got home from the hospital. Her husband is an American and wants very much to be involved in his baby's care, but her mother is from Cuba and sees baby care as her role, and only her role. She even tends to push Juanita aside when it comes to baby care. She also states that she finds many of her mother's ideas old-fashioned, and this is driving her crazy. They all live in a two-bedroom home and the tension is causing problems between Juanita and her husband. "I love my husband, but I can't hurt my mom. I just don't know what to do."

Questions

1. How might the tension between Juanita's mother and husband, and between Juanita and her mother, be affecting Juanita's breastfeeding?

2. How might the problem have been avoided?

3. What suggestions might the nurse give Juanita to relieve the constipation?

4. How will the nurse assess her breastfeeding problems?

5. Are there any community resources that might be helpful for this family?

6. Two days after her delivery, Juanita was given a shot of RhoGAM. At this home visit she asks the nurse why she needed it and if she would have problems with her next pregnancy. How should the nurse reply?

7. Juanita would like to attend a new mothers' group that meets in two weeks. Her mother said that she should not go out for at least 30 days. Juanita is unhappy about this and asks the nurse if she can go. How should the nurse reply?

8. The nurse does an exam on the infant and notices a safety pin on the baby's undershirt with a religious medal on it. What is the significance of this finding?

9. The baby also has a piece of string in the shape of a circle stuck to her forehead. Juanita looks embarrassed when she sees that the nurse notices the string. What is the significance of the string?

10. Juanita tells the nurse that she would like to take a shower and wants to know if it is okay. How should the nurse respond?

Reference

Simpson, K. R., & Creehan, P. A. (2001). *AWHONN perinatal nursing* (2nd ed.). Philadelphia: Lippincott, Williams & Wilkins.

Daphne

AGE

14

SETTING

- Clinic

CULTURAL CONSIDERATIONS

ETHNICITY

- White American

PRE-EXISTING CONDITION

CO-EXISTING CONDITION/CURRENT PROBLEM

- Thyrotoxicosis; BF problems; depression; weight loss; fatigue; palpitations; memory loss; swollen cervical glands

COMMUNICATIONS

DISABILITY

SOCIOECONOMIC STATUS

SPIRITUAL/RELIGIOUS

PSYCHOSOCIAL

- Depression

LEGAL

ETHICAL

PRIORITIZATION

DELEGATION

PHARMACOLOGIC

ALTERNATIVE THERAPY

SIGNIFICANT HISTORY

- Primipara

MODERATE

POSTPARTUM

Level of difficulty: Moderate

Overview: Requires assessing a postpartum woman at three weeks after delivery to rule out thyroid disease.

Client Profile

Daphne is a 14-year-old, SWF, G1P1 who delivered three weeks ago. She is bottle-feeding at this time. Although she had intended to breastfeed, she stopped after two weeks due to sore nipples and concerns about not having enough breast milk.

Case Study

Her mother calls the clinic to report that Daphne seems very moody, depressed, and agitated. She has lost over 10 pounds in one week despite an increased appetite; she complains of headaches, fatigue, palpitations, memory loss, and swollen glands in her neck.

Questions

1. Identify at least three questions the nurse should ask Daphne's mother during this initial phone call.

2. Give three possible explanations for Daphne's symptoms.

3. The nurse tells Daphne's mother to bring her to the clinic for evaluation. The CNM orders a TSH. Why?

4. Which of Daphne's symptoms can be associated with thyroid disease?

5. Her results for her thyroid stimulating hormone (TSH) are 0.24 μIU/mL What is the most probable diagnosis?

6. What additional test will probably be ordered?

7. What are the possible consequences if hyperthyroidism is the problem and it is not diagnosed?

8. Describe the normal involution to be expected for Daphne at this time.

9. What are the most common reasons women decide not to breastfeed after they have started?

10. Daphne states that she is very disappointed that she is not breastfeeding and would like to try to start to breastfeed again. She has bottle-fed for one week now. What is the best response by the nurse?

References

Biancuzzo, M. (2003). *Breastfeeding the newborn: Clinical strategies for nurses* (2nd ed.). St. Louis, MO: Mosby.

Riordan, J., & Auerbach, K. (2005). *Breast feeding and human lactation* (3rd ed.). Sudbury, MA: Jones and Bartlett.

Wheeler, L. (2002). *Nurse-midwifery handbook* (2nd ed.). Philadelphia: Lippincott, Williams & Wilkins.

Sueata

AGE

26

SETTING

- Hospital postpartum unit

CULTURAL CONSIDERATIONS

- Pakistani traditions

ETHNICITY

- Pakistani

PRE-EXISTING CONDITION

CO-EXISTING CONDITION/CURRENT PROBLEM

COMMUNICATIONS

DISABILITY

SOCIOECONOMIC STATUS

- Student

SPIRITUAL/RELIGIOUS

PSYCHOSOCIAL

- No support from fob

LEGAL

ETHICAL

PRIORITIZATION

DELEGATION

PHARMACOLOGIC

ALTERNATIVE THERAPY

SIGNIFICANT HISTORY

- Primigravida

POSTPARTUM

Level of difficulty: Moderate

Overview: Requires an understanding of the Pakistani culture and the low status of women in that culture.

Client Profile

Sueata has been in the United States for four years. She is from a wealthy family in Pakistan. She is on a student visa, which expires in two months. She fell in love with an American student, and he is the father of her baby. They had an argument when she was seven months pregnant, and he has not called her since. She is 26 years old and this was her first pregnancy. The baby is a girl. Sueata is bottle-feeding.

Case Study

Sueata is two days postpartum. She is scheduled for discharge in the morning. The nurse finds her crying quietly, holding her baby in her arms.

Questions

1. The nurse begins to go over discharge instructions with Sueata. Make a list of the routine discharge instructions given to women who have had normal spontaneous vaginal deliveries.

2. Sueata pushes her baby away and cries out, "I hate you. Why couldn't you have been a boy?" How should the nurse respond?

3. Sueata asks about adoption. This is the first time that she has even mentioned that she was thinking about giving her baby up for adoption. How should the nurse approach this subject?

4. Sueata hands the nurse a letter from the immigration service stating that her student visa will expire in two months. Sueata explains through her tears that if she goes home she will be killed. She has dishonored her family by getting pregnant, and they do not want her back. If she goes home, they may even hire someone to kill her. How likely is it that this story may be true? Discuss the status of women in the Pakastani culture.

5. What resources might the nurse offer Sueata?

6. How is childbearing viewed in the Pakastani culture?

7. Will the baby have United States or Pakistani citizenship?

8. What methods of birth control might be acceptable to Sueata?

9. What specific instructions does she need to care for her breasts since she is not breastfeeding?

10. Outline information on formula preparation.

References

Littleton, L., & Engebretson, J. C. (2002). *Maternal, neonatal, and women's health nursing.* Clifton Park, NY: Thomson Delmar Learning.

Ayazlatif, P. (Ed.): (2003). Karo Kari for honour and self pride. *Indus Pak: Resource Center for South Asia and Pakistan.* http://www.31.brinkster.com.

Samya, B. Edited by Regan, E., Brown, R., & Brown, C. (1999). Crime or custom? Violence against women in Pakistan. *Human Rights Watch.* USA.

Roquanda

AGE

24

SETTING

■ Hospital postpartum unit

CULTURAL CONSIDERATIONS

■ Jamician Rastafarian culture

ETHNICITY

■ Black American

PRE-EXISTING CONDITION

■ ML episiotomy; vacuum extractor; Pitocin-augmented labor and birth; epidural anesthesia

CO-EXISTING CONDITION/CURRENT PROBLEM

■ PP hemorrhage

COMMUNICATIONS

DISABILITY

SOCIOECONOMIC STATUS

SPIRITUAL/RELIGIOUS

■ Rastafarian

PSYCHOSOCIAL

LEGAL

ETHICAL

PRIORITIZATION

DELEGATION

PHARMACOLOGIC

■ Hemabate; Pitocin; Methergine

ALTERNATIVE THERAPY

SIGNIFICANT HISTORY

■ Multipara

POSTPARTUM

Level of difficulty: Difficult

Overview: Requires critical thinking to assess, determine cause, and treat a client who experiences postpartum hemorrhage.

DIFFICULT

Client Profile

Roquanda is a 24-year-old, G4P3003, MBF. Her oldest child is 3½ years old. She delivered a 9 pound 12 ounce baby boy following an 18-hour Pitocin-augmented labor with epidural anesthesia this morning. Her second stage was two hours. She was given a mediolateral episiotomy, and the baby's head was delivered by vacuum extractor after she experienced difficulty pushing. Her estimated blood loss (EBL) was 400 mL right after delivery. Immediately after delivery her VS were BP 110/70, temperature 98, pulse 68, and respirations 20. She plans to bottle-feed.

Case Study

Roquanda delivered two hours ago and has just been transferred to the postpartum floor with an IV of lactated ringers, which is to be discontinued when it is finished. Upon assessing her, the postpartum nurse notes that Roquanda is trickling blood from the vagina and has soaked a pad about 30 to 40 minutes after she changes it. Her vital signs are BP 90/68, pulse 100, and respiration 28. She appears restless.

Questions

1. Name three common sources of postpartum hemorrhage. Compare and contrast them according to the signs and symptoms, precipitating factors, and treatment for each.

2. What is the normal expected blood loss for a vaginal delivery?

3. Was Roquanda's blood loss normal?

4. What factors increase the initial blood loss in delivery?

5. List four history factors that increase Roquanda's risk for postpartum hemorrhage.

6. List four labor and delivery factors that increased her risk.

7. Assess her vital signs. Are these normal for postpartum?

8. If not, what is the significance of them?

9. List at least six other signs of shock related to hypovolemia.

10. List at least two consequences of postpartum hemorrhage.

11. Why is Roquanda at an even higher risk for problems related to postpartum hemorrhage?

12. When would you expect Roquanda's hematocrit to be checked? If she had a postpartum hemorrhage, how would you expect it to be reflected in the hematocrit?

13. Roquanda's hematocrit is low, and the certified nurse midwife prescribes iron supplements. The nurse is discharging her on her third postpartum day. What information about taking iron supplements needs to be included in teaching Roquanda?

References

Littleton, L., & Engebretson, J. C. (2002). *Maternal, neonatal, and women's health nursing.* Clifton Park, NY: Thomson Delmar Learning.

Ayazlatif, P. (Ed.): (2003). Karo Kari for honour and self pride. *Indus Pak: Resource Center for South Asia and Pakistan.* http://www.31.brinkster.com.

Samya, B. Edited by Regan, E., Brown, R., & Brown, C. (1999). Crime or custom? Violence against women in Pakistan. *Human Rights Watch.* USA.

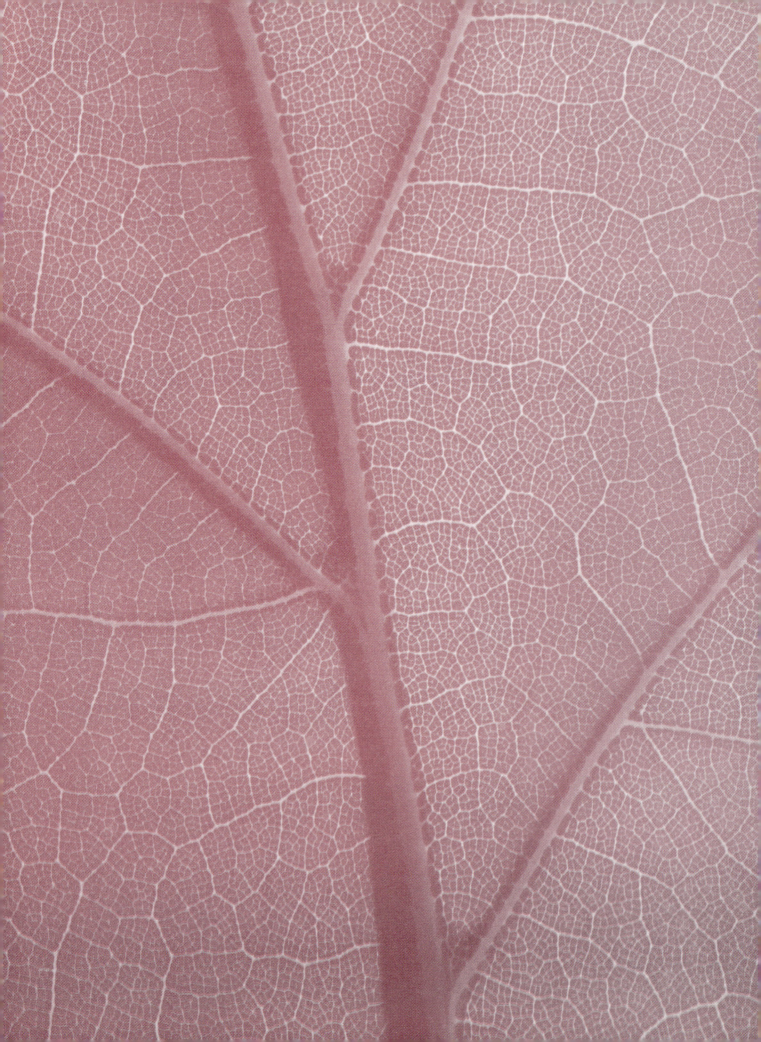

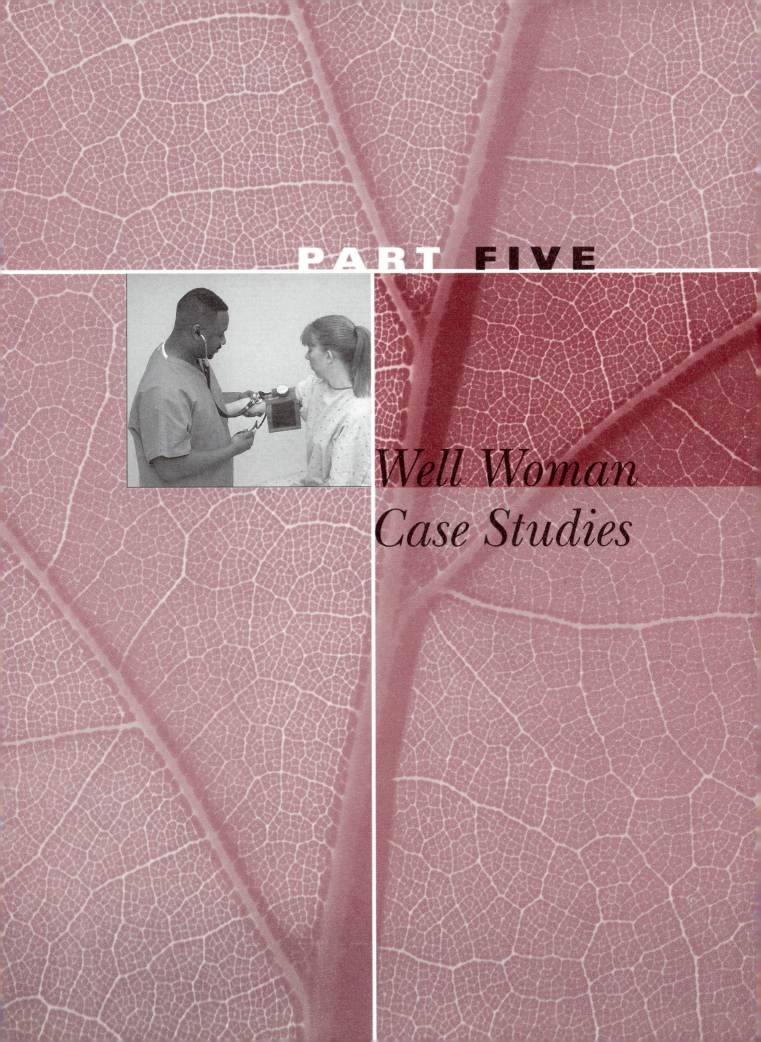

PART FIVE

Well Woman
Case Studies

Carina

AGE

15

SETTING

- Certified Nurse Midwife's office

CULTURAL CONSIDERATIONS

ETHNICITY

- White American

PRE-EXISTING CONDITION

- Anorexia

CO-EXISTING CONDITION/CURRENT PROBLEM

- Primary amenorrhea

COMMUNICATIONS

DISABILITY

SOCIOECONOMIC STATUS

SPIRITUAL/RELIGIOUS

- Baptist

PSYCHOSOCIAL

- Suspected abuse

LEGAL

- Minor

ETHICAL

- Self-determination vs rights of parent

PRIORITIZATION

DELEGATION

PHARMACOLOGIC

ALTERNATIVE THERAPY

SIGNIFICANT HISTORY

WELL WOMAN

Level of difficulty: Easy

Overview: Requires using critical thinking to assess teen for primary amenorrhea. Requires skills in assessing communications with teen regarding sexuality and related risks.

Client Profile

Carina is a 15-year-old, SWF who has been brought to the midwife's office by her mother. She is five feet five inches, and her current weight is 103 pounds. Her mother states that she is not sexually active.

Case Study

Carina's mother expresses concern that Carina has not yet started her menstrual periods. The nurse is taking an initial history and preparing her for the CNM to do her physical exam. Carina indicates that she does not want her mother present for the history and physical. There does not seem to be tension between them, but Carina indicates that she is old enough to be seen alone. Her mother agrees and returns to the waiting room. During the interview Carina is adamant that she is not sexually active. However, after a period of time she does admit to the nurse that she does engage in casual oral sex because it makes her popular. Besides, she does not consider that having sex. She states that she sees nothing wrong with oral sex but would never have intercourse because, "I am not that kind of girl." During the physical exam, the midwife notes that the inner aspects of Carina's arms are bruised and there is an unusual mark on her breast that could be a bite mark. When Carina is questioned about this, she flippantly states that "Oh, that's my boyfriend. He gets a little carried away sometimes."

Questions

1. Since Carina is a minor and does require her mother's consent to have health care, is it necessary for her mother to be present during the history and physical?

2. How does Carina's description of her sexual activity impact the manner in which the nurse will pursue the interview?

3. Does Carina need a PAP smear and/or STI testing?

4. What particular observations will be important for the nurse and the CNM to help determine the cause of her amenorrhea?

5. List five factors that may contribute to the fact that Carina has not yet started her periods.

6. What possible psychosocial impact might this situation have on Carina?

7. Develop a plan for addressing the abuse situation.

8. List four questions specifically intended to explore possible abuse that would be appropriate at this visit.

9. Outline a teaching plan for Carina.

10. Should Carina be offered birth control?

References

Hawkins, J., et al. (1997). *Protocols for nurse practitioners in gynecologic settings* (6th ed.). New York: The Tiresias Press, Inc.

Cyndie

AGE

> 28

SETTING

> ■ Women's clinic

CULTURAL CONSIDERATIONS

ETHNICITY

> ■ Black American

PRE-EXISTING CONDITION

CO-EXISTING CONDITION/CURRENT PROBLEM

> ■ Pelvic inflammatory disease (PID); gonorrhea; chlamydia

COMMUNICATIONS

DISABILITY

SOCIOECONOMIC STATUS

SPIRITUAL/RELIGIOUS

PSYCHOSOCIAL

LEGAL

ETHICAL

PRIORITIZATION

DELEGATION

PHARMACOLOGIC

ALTERNATIVE THERAPY

SIGNIFICANT HISTORY

> ■ Primipara

MODERATE

WELL WOMAN

Level of Difficulty: Moderate

Overview: This case requires that the student use critical thinking to assess and provide care for a client with PID.

Client Profile   **Cyndie** is a 28-year-old, G1P1, MBF. Her first child is six years old. She and her husband have been trying, without success, to conceive for the past four years. Her first pregnancy was completely normal, and the baby was delivered via a normal spontaneous vaginal delivery at a birth center. Cyndie works as a television announcer.

Case Study   Cyndie is being seen today at the Women's clinic with a vaginal discharge, pelvic pain, and a fever of 101.6°F. A pregnancy test is negative. She has a purulent, irritating vaginal discharge, feels nauseated all the time, and has dysuria.

Questions

1. What test should the nurse anticipate?

2. The client is diagnosed with gonorrhea. What other infection is commonly found with gonorrhea?

3. Just after her last baby was born Cyndie was diagnosed with gonorrhea/chlamydia infections and treated. How might these infections leave her with secondary infertility?

4. Cyndie does not have any drug allergies. What is the most common treatment for these infections?

5. Should she be re-screened? If so, when?

6. Is the clinician required to report these diseases to the public health department? If yes, how is this done?

7. Cyndie also complains of pain around the opening of her vagina on the right side. On inspection the clinician finds an enlarged glandular lump around 2 cm in diameter. This is most probably what?

8. Cyndie also jumps when the clinician moves her cervix. What conditions is cervical motion tenderness (Chandelier's sign) associated with?

9. Outline the teaching the nurse needs to provide to Cyndie prior to her leaving the office today.

10. If Cyndie were pregnant, how would her treatment be different?

Reference

MMWR. (2002). http://www.cdc.gov/std/treatment/default.htm.

Varney, H., Kriebs, J., & Gegor, C. (2004). *Varney's midwifery* (4th ed.). Sudbury, MA: Jones & Bartlett.

Anna

AGE

36

SETTING

■ Well Woman clinic

CULTURAL CONSIDERATIONS

ETHNICITY

■ Black American

PRE-EXISTING CONDITION

CO-EXISTING CONDITION/CURRENT PROBLEM

■ Breast lump; fatigue

COMMUNICATIONS

DISABILITY

SOCIOECONOMIC STATUS

SPIRITUAL/RELIGIOUS

PSYCHOSOCIAL

LEGAL

ETHICAL

PRIORITIZATION

DELEGATION

PHARMACOLOGIC

■ Oral contraceptive pills (OCP)

ALTERNATIVE THERAPY

SIGNIFICANT HISTORY

■ Multipara

WELL WOMAN

Level of difficulty: Moderate

Overview: Requires critical thinking to differentiate signs associated with benign breast disease from those associated with serious breast lumps.

Client Profile

Anna is a 36-year-old, G4P4, MBF. Anna just moved to Miami three months ago. She is using OCPs for contraception. She has a 10-year-old son and three daughters ages 9, 7, and 4. She breastfed all of her children for at least a year. She is active in all of her children's activities. She is a baseball coach, helps at the junior high in the book store, is on the PTSA (parent teacher student association) planning committee, and keeps the books for her husband's business. Lately she has been feeling more tired than usual.

Case Study

Anna is being seen at the Well Woman clinic for her annual exam. She is actually six months overdue, but last week when doing a breast self-exam she noticed a small lump in her right breast. There were no dimpling or retractions noted on the breast.

Questions

1. What is the significance of the fact that Anna breastfed all of her children for at least a year each?

2. What screening and diagnostic tests are appropriate for Anna at this visit?

3. Anna describes the lump as very small, having irregular edges and not painful. Any clinically palpable mass requires further assessment. What type of lump commonly presents with these characteristics?

4. The nurse examines Anna and finds the lump is fixed and located in the outer upper quadrant of the breast. Are these additional findings reassuring or non-reassuring?

5. The nurse also notices no scaling or nipple discharge and no infraclavicular or supraclavicular adenopathy. However, she did note edema in the auxiliary area of Anna's right arm. What is the significance of this?

6. Which screening test for breast cancer is most appropriate to start with for Anna—an ultrasound or a mammogram?

7. If the mammogram reveals a suspicious lump, what will be the next step to diagnosis if it is cancer?

8. Give at least two possible causes of Anna's fatigue that are not related to the breast lump.

9. List at least three questions that the nurse needs to ask Anna to help determine the cause of her fatigue.

10. Identify two community resources that can offer support to Anna and her family if the breast lump is cancerous.

11. Are Black women more or less at risk for breast cancer?

References

HHS Affirms value of mammogram for detection of breast cancer. (2002). HHS Release, U.S. Dept. of Health and Human Services.

Littleton, L., & Engbretson, J. (2002). *Maternal, neonatal and women's health nursing.* Clifton Park, NY: Thomson Delmar Learning.

Morgan, G., & Hamilton, C. (2003). *Practice guidelines for obstetrics and gynecology* (2nd ed.). Philadelphia: Lippincott, Williams & Wilkins.

Jodi

AGE

31

SETTING

- Certified Nurse Midwife's office

CULTURAL CONSIDERATIONS

ETHNICITY

- Hispanic American

PRE-EXISTING CONDITION

CO-EXISTING CONDITION/CURRENT PROBLEM

- Abnormal PAP; condylomata acuminata human papillomavirus; gonorrhea; chlamydia

COMMUNICATIONS

DISABILITY

SOCIOECONOMIC STATUS

SPIRITUAL/RELIGIOUS

PSYCHOSOCIAL

LEGAL

ETHICAL

PRIORITIZATION

DELEGATION

PHARMACOLOGIC

- Flagyl; 2.5% Nupercainal ointment; doxycycline; erythromycin; azithromycin; ofloxicin; ceftriaxone; cefotaxime; spectinomycin; ciprofloxacin; alendronate (Fosamax); raloxifen (Evista)
- HRT therapy; Depo-Provera; clonidine; trichloroacetic acid (TCA); podophyllin; 5-FU or imiquimod cream

ALTERNATIVE THERAPY

- Black cohosh

SIGNIFICANT HISTORY

- Multipara

MODERATE

WELL WOMAN

Level of difficulty: Moderate

Overview: Requires the student to use critical thinking to assess a client who has an abnormal PAP and to provide education for that client.

Client Profile

Jodi is a 31-year-old G2P2, MHF. She works full time as a high school algebra teacher. Her two children are 7 and 8 years old. She is five feet three inches, and her weight is 112 pounds. She does not want any more children and her current birth control is the contraceptive patch.

Family History: Both of Jodi's parents are alive and well. She has two sisters who are also alive and well. Her maternal grandfather died of a heart attack at age 62. Her other grandparents are all still alive and well.

Medical/Surgical History: Benign

OB/GYN History: She has had two full term normal spontaneous deliveries. Both babies were healthy and appropriately grown (AGA). Prior to her first baby she had a routine PAP smear that was ASCUS with atypia favoring inflammation. This was determined to be bacterial vaginosis, and she was treated with Flagyl. Her next two PAP smears after that were normal. Then during her second pregnancy, she had a routine PAP smear done, which showed ASCUS with atypia now favoring HPV infection. Acetic acid 5% was swabbed on the cervix and several small areas turned white. She was asymptomatic and there were no changes in the lesions throughout the pregnancy. After delivery she returned for a normal postpartum visit and another repeat PAP smear, which again showed ASCUS with atypia favoring HPV; she was sent for a colposcopy and was successfully treated with cryotherapy with complete resolution. After the cryotherapy her repeat PAP smears were all normal. She was told that no more follow-up would be needed since her PAP smears have all been normal since.

Case Study

It has been seven years since her abnormal PAPs. Jodi is now being seen in the office today for her annual exam and a routine repeat PAP test. During the exam the CNM noticed a small external venereal wart present on the inner surface of the labia. A vaginal cervical exam revealed some slight acteowhite cervical changes present. A PAP smear and DNA probe for gonorrhea and chlamydia were done. Local treatment was started with topical podophyllin solution to the wart.

The current repeat PAP smear came back showing high-grade sqamous interepithelial lesion (HGSIL) with high-grade SIL changes. She was sent for a colposcopy, and the biopsy showed severe cervical dysplasia favoring carcinoma in situ. The DNA probe was positive for both gonorrhea and chlamydia, and she was treated. The CNM tried to do some patient counseling with Jodi, but she was totally distraught and was angrily going to confront her husband, who denied having any affairs. She told the CNM that she has been totally faithful to her husband and does not understand how she could have gotten these diseases. She asks if it is possible that she got them at the high school swimming pool where she has been taking her children to swim on the weekends.

Questions

1. Discuss HPV infections.

2. If a client complains of discomfort associated with the HPV treatment, what suggestions can the nurse give her for pain relief?

3. How should the nurse respond to Jodi's question about the swimming pool?

4. Since this last PAP came back showing high-grade SIL changes, what treatment should the nurse anticipate that Jodi will be referred for?

5. What is the significance of the different grades of different PAP smear abnormalities?

6. What is the significance of and treatment for gonorrhea and chlamydia?

7. Jodi says she is tired of using birth control and asks the nurse about permanent sterilization. How should the nurse reply?

8. What are the clinical consequences of a premature surgical hysterectomy?

9. What are the different treatment options available for these types of cutaneous lesion?

10. What type of continuing patient instructions and follow-up will be needed?

11. Will the partner need to be treated for any of the infections?

References

Bethesda 2001 Terminology. www.bethesda2001.cancer.gov.

Choma, K. (2003). ASC-US and HPV testing. *American Journal of Nursing, 103*(2), 42–50.

Morgan, G., & Hamilton, C. (2003). *Practice guidelines for obstetrics and gynecology.* Philadelphia: Lippincott, Williams & Wilkins.

CDCP 2002. *STD treatment guidelines.* www.cdc.gov.

Jing

AGE

36

SETTING

- Infertility specialty center

CULTURAL CONSIDERATIONS

- Shinto health beliefs

ETHNICITY

- Asian American

PRE-EXISTING CONDITION

- Dysmenorrhea; dyspareunia; increasingly irregular menses; chronic pelvic pain

CO-EXISTING CONDITION/CURRENT PROBLEM

- Endometriosis; infertility; strangulated right ovary

COMMUNICATIONS

DISABILITY

SOCIOECONOMIC STATUS

- IVF is very expensive

SPIRITUAL/RELIGIOUS

- IVF procedures/options; Shinto

PSYCHOSOCIAL

- Stress secondary to reproductive disturbance

LEGAL

ETHICAL

- Destruction of embryo vs ability to carry to viability

PRIORITIZATION

DELEGATION

PHARMACOLOGIC

- Clomiphene citrate (Clomid); Lupron; Synarel

ALTERNATIVE THERAPY

- Accupuncture

SIGNIFICANT HISTORY

- Nulligravida; dysmenorrhea; dyspareunia; increasing irregular menses; chronic pelvic pain

WELL WOMAN

Level of difficulty: Moderate

Overview: Requires understanding endometriosis and its effects on fertility and Shinto health belief system.

Client Profile

Jing is a 36-year-old, G0, married, Asian female who has been previously seen in the clinic for an infertility workup and treatment. She has been having unprotected sexual intercourse for the past 24 months without any conception to date. Her gynecological history includes a history of dysmenorrhea, dyspareunia, increasingly irregular menses, and chronic pelvic pain. Her OBGYN history includes menses onset at nine years old. Her periods are from 24 to 28 days with a 9- to 11-day flow using 5 to 6 pads the first day. A basic introductory history and physical examination were completed. She had some basic lab work drawn and was given an infertility diary to fill out before her next visit.

Case Study

Two weeks later she was seen in the emergency room with high fever, nausea, vomiting, and severe right lower quadrant abdominal pain. She is stoic in her response to pain. Her CBC showed a leukocytosis with a mild bandemia and urine analysis with moderate blood and trace protein. Pelvic ultrasound showed a moderate size pelvic mass in the appendical/tuboovarian region. After a diagnosis of an acute appendicitis was made, she was taken to the operating room. Exploration of the right lower quadrant revealed a strangulated right ovary suspended from a twisted necrotic fallopian tube and diffuse adhesions from the diffuse generalized endometriosis present throughout the right pelvis and abdomen. The surgeons need to perform a right oophorectomy, appendectomy, and adhesion analysis. During the surgery the surgeons also performed some laser coagulation on the numerous endometriosis lesions that were present on the uterus, colon, deep peritoneum, cul-de-sac, omentum, and ipsilateral ovary. Since discharge she has done well and is now here for a six-week postoperative check.

Questions

1. What is endometriosis, and how does it affect the health of the women who develop the disorder?

2. What are the classic signs and symptoms?

3. What is the natural course of endometriosis?

4. What are the different risk factors for the development of endometriosis?

5. What are the different treatment options available for endometriosis?

6. What are chocolate cysts, and how are they treated?

7. Does endometriosis cause cancer?

8. Identify several resources that the nurse can refer Jing to for support.

9. Describe how endometriosis is staged.

10. Are there any natural treatments that have been successful in reducing pain from endometriosis?

References

Daiter, E. (2004). *Infertility tutorials.* Coastal Publications, LLC. http://www.infertilitytutorials.com/index.cfm.

Northrup, C. (1998). *Women's bodies, women's wisdom.* New York: Bantam Books.

Sills, E. S., Perole, M., Stamm, L. J., Kaplan, C. R., & Tucker, M. J. (2004). Medical and psychological management of recurrent abortion, history of postneonatal death, ectopic pregnancy and infertility: Successful implementation of IVF for multifactorial reproductive dysfunction. A case report. *Clinical & Experimental Obstetrics & Gynecology* 31(2):143–146.

Sylvia

AGE

- 48

SETTING

- Well Women private clinic

CULTURAL CONSIDERATIONS

- Black American professional culture

ETHNICITY

- Black American

PRE-EXISTING CONDITION

- Perimenopause; hypertension

CO-EXISTING CONDITION/CURRENT PROBLEM

- Hypothyroidism; pituitary tumor; obesity; tobacco use; occasional alcohol use

COMMUNICATIONS

DISABILITY

SOCIOECONOMIC STATUS

- Professional

SPIRITUAL/RELIGIOUS

PSYCHOSOCIAL

- Cares for aging mother; work/life balance issues

LEGAL

ETHICAL

PRIORITIZATION

DELEGATION

PHARMACOLOGIC

- Atenolol; fluoxetine (Prozac); calcium; vitamin D

ALTERNATIVE THERAPY

- St. John's wort

SIGNIFICANT HISTORY

- Primipara

WELL WOMAN

Level of difficulty: Moderate

Overview: This case requires that the student be able to assess clinical findings to identify a client with hypothyroidism and potential pituitary tumor. The student is also asked to review prescription medications and possible interactions with the over-the-counter self-medications a client is taking. Finally the student is asked to formulate a care plan complete with teaching.

Client Profile

Sylvia is a 48-year-old, G1P0101, MBF. Her only son is 28 years old and lives in another state. He is married with his own family, and although she is close to her son, they only see each other once a year at Christmas. They do call each other weekly. She has two grandchildren who visit her in the summers for a week. She is divorced and lives with her mother. Her mother suffered a severe stroke ten years ago and she needs assistance with her daily care. During the hours Sylvia works, she has a nursing assistant stay with her mother. After work she assumes full responsibility for caring for her mother. Sylvia is a registered nurse. Currently she is the vice president in charge of nursing at a large teaching hospital. She has 25 years of nursing experience and up until the past two years has been known as a dynamic hands-on leader. Two years ago she experienced a small stroke, which has slowed her down considerably. Although she fully recovered from the stroke, she has found that she no longer has the energy she used to have. She has also gained considerable weight since her stroke. She is five feet three inches tall and her current weight is 168 pounds (BMI 29.8). Sylvia smokes approximately two packs a day and drinks an occasional beer in the late afternoon to relax.

Case Study

Sylvia presents at the Well Woman clinic today for her annual checkup. Her current complaints include lack of energy, noticeable hair loss, weight gain, irregular (every 2 or 3 months) very heavy periods that up until about eight months ago were fairly regular and fairly light, swelling in her feet and ankles at night, and decreasing ability to concentrate. She has started to get headaches that last for several hours and occur at least twice a week. She is not sexually active. She does breast self-exams and states that she has not felt anything unusual, but is worried about a blackish green discharge from her right nipple. After talking to the nurse for a short time she also admits to bouts of depression, which are lasting longer and longer. At today's visit the nurse notes the following: BP 156/88, P 88, R 20; thyroid gland palpable with bruit; skin dry; hair coarse and nails brittle. At her last visit she was prescribed atenolol 50 mg daily to manage her hypertension and fluoxetine (Prozac) 20 mg daily for mild depression.

In an attempt to avoid osteoporosis she takes calcium 1200 mg (600 mg in the morning and 600 mg in the evening) with vitamin D. Because her depression has been getting worse, she also started to take St John's wort 900 mg divided into three doses daily.

Questions

1. Identify at least three possible reasons for Sylvia's weight gain.

2. Make a list of the lab tests that the nurse should anticipate will be ordered for Sylvia at this visit.

3. Give four possible causes for her fatigue.

4. Sylvia has yearly mammograms, does breast self-exams, gets a yearly complete physical, and has no family history of cancer. Using the data from her profile and the case study, assess her risks for breast cancer.

5. How does Sylvia's lifestyle contribute to her chances of having another stroke?

6. How common is thyroid disease in women?

7. Assess her risks for cardiovascular disease.

8. Assess her menstrual changes.

9. Analyze the following lab results:

Cholesterol:
LDL 146 mg/dL
VLDL 41 mg/dL
HDL 33 mg/dL
Triglycerides 207 mg/dL
Total cholesterol 220 mg/dL
TSH 10.2 µIU/mL

10. Sylvia is a Black American woman. How might her race impact on her health risk factors?

11. Many women will self-medicate with over-the-counter medications, herbals, etc. Review her prescription medications and her self-medication and comment on any interactions she needs to be made aware of.

References

Overweight prevalence. (2000). http://www.cdc.gov/nchs/fastats/overwt.htm.

Wheeler, L. (2002). *Nurse-midwifery handbook* (2nd ed.). Philadelphia: Lippincott, Williams & Wilkins.

Whitneye, N., Cataldo, C. B., & Rolfer, S. R. (2002). *Understanding normal and clinical nutrition.* Belmont, CA: Thompson/Wadsworth Learning.

Thyroid through the ages: Midlife (menopause). http://www.aace.com/pub/tam2001/tam-midlife.php.

Risk factors. http://www.nuff.org/health_riskfactors.htm.

JNC-VII report on management of hypertension. http://hp2010.nhlbihin.net.

Josephine

AGE

68

SETTING

- Well Woman clinic

CULTURAL CONSIDERATIONS

- Advanced age

ETHNICITY

- White American

PRE-EXISTING CONDITION

- Malnutrition; asthma

CO-EXISTING CONDITION/CURRENT PROBLEM

- Osteoporosis

COMMUNICATIONS

- Not communicating needs with children

DISABILITY

SOCIOECONOMIC STATUS

- Poverty

SPIRITUAL/RELIGIOUS

- Catholic

PSYCHOSOCIAL

- Isolation

LEGAL

ETHICAL

PRIORITIZATION

DELEGATION

PHARMACOLOGIC

- HRT

ALTERNATIVE THERAPY

SIGNIFICANT HISTORY

- Multipara; surgical menopause—HRT × 5 years; *Family history:* Heart disease, breast cancer, Alzheimer's disease, and osteoporosis; tobacco use for 20 years

WELL WOMAN

Level of difficulty: Difficult

Overview: Requires knowledge base concerning hormone replacement therapy and menopausal risk for osteoporosis. This case looks at common economic problems facing older woman.

DIFFICULT

Client Profile

Josephine is a 68-year-old, G3P3003, widowed, white female. She breastfed all of her children for one year. Her last physical exam was three years ago. At that time she was five feet, five inches tall and weighed 110 lbs.

Family History: Mother died of a heart attack at age 82; father is living but has Alzheimer's and is living in a complete care facility. She has two sisters; one is 72 and is very healthy except for some minor problems with osteoporosis, and the other one is 76 and is fighting the final stages of breast cancer. She takes short walks, but lately she has been afraid to walk alone since there have been some muggings of older people in her neighborhood. Her children have encouraged her to come live with them to get away from her changing neighborhood, but she has many good memories of her husband there and does not want to leave her home. Besides, she does not want to become a burden to her children. She has a dog, who is now 12 years old, and a cat, 13 years old, as her only companions. She is very attached to her pets.

Medical History: Asthma as a child and into the teens. She smoked one pack of cigarettes a day for 20 years, but quit 14 years ago, when she could not afford it anymore.

Surgical History: Hysterectomy and oophorectomy at age 48 for menometrorrhagia. She took HRT for five years for hot flashes and mood swings and then decided to discontinue them herself.

Psychosocial History: She is living on a diminishing income. Her husband died four years ago after a long fight with lung cancer. With his death, her income dropped to half. She has Medicare but cannot afford the supplemental coverage. Her children do not know how financially needy she is, and she will not tell them. She says, "They all have children in college and they need their money." Some days she is only able to eat one meal and often that meal is a bowl of cereal. She does make sure that her pets eat each day.

Case Study

Today Josephine is being seen in the Well Woman clinic for progressively worsening backache. On exam her height is five feet three inches and her weight is 106 pounds.

Questions

1. Identify at least three health risks for Josephine and give at least two pieces of supporting data for each of your choices.

2. How does her history of breastfeeding for three years affect her risk for osteoporosis?

3. How does breastfeeding affect her risk for breast cancer today?

4. Define menometrorrhagia.

5. Does Josephine need a PAP smear today?

6. What other screening tests are appropriate for her at this visit?

7. How does surgical menopause differ from natural menopause?

8. What effect does her five years on HRT have on her health risk for heart disease?

9. What effect does her five years on HRT have on her health risk for osteoporosis?

10. What resources can you suggest to help with her financial and living situation?

11. Develop a teaching plan to help Josephine minimize her health risk.

References

Morgan, G., & Hamilton, C. (2003). *Practice guidelines for obstetrics and gynecology* (2nd ed.). Philadelphia: Lippincott, Williams & Wilkins.

Whitney, N., Cataldo, C. B., & Rolfer, S. R. (2002). *Understanding normal and clinical nutrition.* Belmont, CA: Thompson/Wadsworth Learning.

Answers

Part 1: Prenatal Case Studies

Case Study 1:   *Linda*

1. **"I am worried about these bumps on my nipples, and why are my breasts so tender?"** Linda has noticed that the Montgomery tubercles on her areolae have gotten larger. These sebaceous glands provide nipple lubrication and antisepsis. The most important thing to teach Linda about them is that they are normal and that she should not wash her areolae and nipples with soap. Soap will dry the nipples and may cause cracking later when she breastfeeds her baby. The tenderness is probably due to the effects of estrogen preparing the breast for lactation later. It causes proliferation and differentiation of the ductal system. Progesterone also promotes an increase in the lobes and lobules and alveoli. Adrenocorticotropic hormone (ACTH) with growth hormone and prolactin and progesterone promote growth. All of these changes may cause tenderness of the breast.

2. **"Look at this line on my abdomen; where did that come from and what is the brownish coloring on my face?"** The dark line running from her umbilicus to the pubic bone is called the linea nigra. The darker areas on her face, called chloasma or melasma gravidarum, are the result of increased estrogen, progesterone, and α-melanocytic stimulating hormone. These are normal pigmentation changes in pregnancy usually seen more in women with dark hair.

3. **"Is it going to always be there?"** In most cases the hyperpigmentation that occurs in pregnancy will fade during the postpartum. However, in some women with darker skin and hair, it may remain. Linda should be taught to stay out of the sun, as the sun will exacerbate the hyperpigmentation.

4. **"I have this vaginal discharge. It doesn't itch or smell bad, but I notice I am a lot wetter than I have ever been before."** The most likely cause of this increase is that it is a normal change. This increased discharge is one of the body's ways of protecting the mother and fetus from infection. It is called leucorrhea and is thick, white, and acidotic. It discourages colonization of the vagina with harmful organisms. It is important to rule out other possible causes of discharge. Some common causes of abnormal vaginal discharge in pregnancy are bacterial vaginosis (BV), trichomoniasis, and candidiasis. These can be ruled out by examining the discharge via a wet mount, checking the pH, and a "whiff test." Both bacterial vaginosis and trichomoniasis are malodorous. Candidiasis is a fungal infection and does not have an odor. A whiff test is done by putting a drop of the discharge on a slide and adding potassium hydroxide to the slide. If there is a strong fishy odor, the test is considered to be positive; this would

147

most likely indicate bacterial vaginosis, although trichomoniasis may also produce the same results. Bacterial vaginosis will also contain clue cells that can be seen under a microscope prepared in a saline base. The discharge clings to the sides of the vagina and has a grayish color. The motile parasitic protozoan Trichomonas organisms can be seen under the microscope. Trichomonas discharge tends to be frothy and greenish in color. BV and trichomoniasis are both treated with metronidazole (Flagyl) after the first trimester. Untreated, they may increase the woman's risk for preterm labor. Finally gonorrhea and chlamydia may also produce a discharge and should be ruled out.

5. **What is Linda's gravida/para?** This is Linda's third pregnancy. Her gravida is three. Since she carried one baby past 20 weeks and had one termination during the first trimester, her para would be listed at 0 for no full-term pregnancies, 1 for the preterm baby, 1 for the abortion, and 0 for living children or 0110. Therefore she is a G3P0110.

6. **Linda is very excited because her due date is on her birthday. She asks the nurse how certain it is that the baby will actually be born on that date. How should the nurse respond?** The nurse needs to explain that due dates are estimates. Only about 5% of women actually deliver on their due dates. The baby will probably be born anywhere from two weeks prior to the date to up to two weeks after the date.

7. **Linda admits that maybe she did miss a birth control pill several months ago. She continued to take them up to the day she saw her family doctor about the nausea and vomiting and found out she was pregnant. She asks the nurse how dangerous this might be to the baby she is carrying. How should the nurse reply?** While taking hormones during pregnancy is not recommended and there is a potential risk to the fetus, continuing birth control pills has not been demonstrated in studies to be a problem. Many women have not been aware of a pregnancy and continued to take birth control pills without effects to their babies. There are a few long-term studies that have looked at the growth and development of infants born to women who had taken oral contraceptive pills in early pregnancy. They do not show adverse effects. There is one study that suggests that these infants are more prone to urinary tract problems (Li De-Kun, 1995). If she is concerned, she can be referred for genetic counseling.

8. **Besides ultrasound, how can a due date be identified when there is no regular and accurate menstrual history to rely on?** The due date can be estimated by looking at subjective signs such as the first time she feels the baby move (quickening). For most women this will be at about 16 to 22 weeks. The fundal height may also be used to estimate the due date. At 20 weeks the fundal height is usually at the umbilicus. If Linda's baby is growing properly, her fundal height would be halfway between the symphysis pubis and the umbilicus at this visit.

9. **Linda asks the nurse when she can first expect to feel her baby move. What is the best response by the nurse?** Most women will first feel fetal movements between 16 and 22 weeks. Women expecting their first baby (primigravidas) usually feel movement later than those who have experienced pregnancy before (multigravidas). **What is this movement called?** The first movements felt by the mother are called quickening.

10. **Everything is normal at this initial visit. When should the nurse schedule Linda to return for her next prenatal visit?** Linda will be scheduled to return for her next prenatal visit in four weeks. After 28 weeks she will come every two weeks until the 36th week, and then she will be seen weekly. The U.S. Public Health Service recommends that primigravidas be seen initially between six and eight weeks, then again in four weeks. The third visit should be between 14 and 16 weeks and the fourth visit between 24 and 28 weeks. The fifth visit should be at 32 weeks and sixth at 36 weeks. The seventh visit should be at 38 weeks, eighth at 40 weeks, and ninth at 41 weeks. A mulitgravida without complications can be seen less frequently. The recommended schedule for them is again first visit between six and eight weeks, second between 14 and 16 weeks, and third between 24 and 26 weeks. The fifth visit should be at 35 weeks, sixth at 39 weeks and seventh at 41 weeks. These schedules allow for testing at specific points in the pregnancy when potential complications are most likely to be identified.

11. **Identify at least three areas of education that the nurse needs to address at this initial visit.** There are many areas to cover. Linda needs to review her diet and receive instruction on balancing her intake and avoiding long periods of not eating. Pregnant women are prone to hypoglycemia, which is not healthy for the baby and may increase the mother's nausea and vomiting. She should be taught about safety, including using both lap and shoulder seat belts when traveling in a car, and the safe way to exercise without jerking and pulling movements. Due to the hormone changes in pregnancy, the woman is at risk of pulling ligaments and injuring herself. The nurse should review hazards that Linda should avoid including smoking, secondhand smoke, any over-the-counter or prescription drugs not prescribed by the midwife, as well as noxious fumes and chemicals that may be found in her environment. The nurse needs to answer her questions and provide anticipatory guidance on what she can expect in the period from this visit to the next. Since Linda was concerned about the vaginal discharge, it is important that the nurse advise her not to douche. Linda will probably be offered screening tests for abnormalities at the next visit. The nurse should give her literature to take home and read about the tests so that she can make an informed decision about having the tests, or declining the tests, at the next visit. Screening tests may identify normal infants as having potential genetic defects. This adds stress to a pregnancy and may lead to invasive testing, which may result in the loss of the infant. The need and/or desire for such testing needs to be individually decided by the mother. Factors which appear to be most significant in the decision to test or not to test are correlated closely to the mother's attitudes about Down syndrome and fetal loss, rather than her age or racial/ethnic and socioeconomic association. The testing that identifies the most Down syndrome babies, with the lowest false positive rates, involves using an integrated test that consists of nuchal translucency and pregnancy associated plasma protein-A (PAPP-A) at 11 completed weeks of pregnancy, and alpha-fetoprotein, unconjugated estriol (uE(3)), free beta or total human chorionic gonadotropin (hCG), and inhibin-A in the early second trimester.

References

Blackburn, S. (2003). *Maternal, fetal and neonatal physiology* (2nd ed.). St Louis, MO: W. B. Saunders Co.

Kuppermann, M., Nease, R. F., Jr., Gates, E., Learman, L. A., Blumberg, B., Gildengorin, V., et al. (2004, June). How do women of diverse backgrounds value prenatal testing outcomes? *Prenat Diagn., 24*(6), 424–429.

Li, De-Kun, Daling, J. R., Mueller, B. A., Hickok, D. E., Fantel, A. G., & Weiss, N. S. (1995). Oral contraceptives use after conception in relation to the risk of congenital urinary tract anomalies. *Teratology, 51,* 30–36.

Wald, N. J., Rodeck, C., Hackshaw, A. K., & Rudnicka, A. (2004, June). SURUSS in perspective. *BJOG: An International Journal of Obstetrics & Gynaecology 111*(6): 521–531.

Wheeler, L. (2002). *Nurse-midwifery handbook* (2nd ed.). Philadelphia: Lippincott, Williams & Wilkins.

Case Study 2:   *Aries*

1. **If Aries had a 28-day cycle, when is the baby due?** (7 − 3 = 4; 6 + 7 = 13) Her due date is April 13.

2. **How many weeks gestation is she today?** Today she is 19-4/7 weeks gestation.

3. **What is the possible reason why the nurse is having a problem getting a history from Aries and/or her grandmother regarding Aries?** Native Americans tend to be present oriented. This means that they do not see the relevance of the past to current events (Simpson, 2002).

4. **What is the significance of the grandmother bringing Aries to the initial prenatal visit?** Native Americans are respectful of elders, who generally take charge of decision making within a family (Simpson, 2002).

5. **How can the nurse obtain a better estimate of how much Aries drinks?** The nurse can use open-ended questions that are not judgmental. "Tell me about a typical weekend when you go out with your friends." Then narrow it down to what types of drinks and how many.

6. **How much weight should Aries gain in the pregnancy?** Between 20 and 25 pounds would be a good amount. Aries is slightly overweight for her height now, but since she is a teen and is still growing, she needs to gain an adequate amount for the pregnancy. Most important is how she gains the weight and the quality of the food she eats. The ideal weight gain is three to five pounds in the first trimester and then one pound a week for the rest of the pregnancy.

7. **List at least three risk factors associated with Aries's pregnancy.**
   - Teen alcohol use
   - Tobacco use
   - Poverty
   - Late entry into care

8. **Aries's grandmother instructs her to take herbs to improve her blood, but her sister (a nursing student) wants her to take iron supplements. Which advice do you think Aries will follow? Why?** She will follow the advice her grandmother gives since the grandmother is perceived as the head of the house.

9. **Aries decides to quit school at 20 weeks gestation and stay close to home. She spends more time with her grandmother listening to stories while her grandmother works on quilts and macramé. They do not make anything for the baby. Why?** Some Native Americans believe that it is not wise to prepare things for the baby because that could bring harm to the baby.

10. **Aries is forbidden from working on the macramé. Why?** Some Native Americans believe that tying knots can cause knots in the umbilical cord.

11. **Give two common mistakes that nurses make when trying to provide care to women from cultures they are not familiar with.**
    ■ Generalizing some beliefs or traditions to the entire population
    ■ Not looking at the whole picture: some behaviors/beliefs are linked to culture, others to poverty, etc.

References

Littleton, L., & Engebretson, J. C. (2002). *Maternal, neonatal, and women's health nursing.* Clifton Park, NY: Thomson Delmar Learning.

Simpson, K. R., & Creehan, P. A. (2001). *AWHONN perinatal nursing* (2nd ed.). Philadelphia: Lippincott, Williams & Wilkins.

Case Study 3:

Fayola

1. **What are the most common reasons for backaches at 24 wga?** The most common causes are related to the enlarging uterus and are a result of pulling on the stretched ligaments. The round ligament will cause groin pain and the broad and ileosacrum ligament will cause backache. These are made worse by poor posture and high-heel shoes. Braxton Hicks contractions may also cause backache. Pyelonephritis may present as a backache. Finally, preterm labor may present as intermittent backaches and must be ruled out.

2. **List at least five questions the nurse needs to ask Fayola about her backache to begin to assess the necessity of her coming to the clinic at this time.**
    ■ Does she have any vaginal discharge or spotting?
    ■ Are the backaches constant or intermittent? If they are intermittent, has she timed them?
    ■ Does the backache go away when she walks around, or if she lies down?
    ■ Does the pain radiate to her lower abdomen?
    ■ If it is determined that she is having contractions, how strong are they?
    ■ Does she have signs or symptoms of kidney infections, including chills, fever, and/or nausea and vomiting?
    ■ Has she taken antihistamines lately?

3. **What are Braxton Hicks contractions?** These are contractions of the uterus not related to labor.

4. **Is it common for women expecting their first babies to have uncomfortable Braxton Hicks contractions at this time in their pregnancies?** No. Although Braxton Hicks contractions are the most common reason for contractions in the later half of pregnancy, they are usually not uncomfortable at this time and careful assessment must be made to rule out preterm labor.

5. **What are the typical characteristics of Braxton Hicks contractions?**
    ■ Irregular
    ■ Usually not painful
    ■ Usually feel like the baby is "balling up" in the front; seldom do they involve the back

- They stop with activity change
- They do not change the cervix
- They are not accompanied by increased vaginal discharge

6. **What advice can the nurse give Fayola if she believes that the contractions are Braxton Hicks?** If Fayola was resting when she felt the contractions, she should get up and walk around. Braxton Hicks contractions will stop with a change in activity. The nurse should also advise her to drink at least 8 to 10 glasses of water a day. Dehydration may cause uterine irritability. If her contractions are every 10 to 15 minutes apart, if after an hour and after drinking several glasses of water they do not go away, if she experiences any increase in vaginal discharge with or without bleeding, or if she feels pressure like the baby is pushing down, Fayola needs to be brought into the clinic for evaluation and to rule out preterm labor.

7. **If the nurse suspects preterm labor, what should she advise Fayola to do?** The nurse should advise her to go to the hospital or clinic for evaluation immediately.

8. **Fayola goes to the hospital where her contractions are timed at being 30 to 40 seconds and coming every ten minutes. What further evaluation will be done to confirm if these are labor or Braxton Hicks contractions?**
   - She will be given fluids either by IV or orally to hydrate her.
   - A sterile speculum exam will be done to assess for ruptured membranes and to assess the cervix.
   - External fetal and uterine monitoring will be done to evaluate the contraction pattern.
   - A wet mount will be done to assess for vaginal infections and possibly cultures will be taken for STI evaluation.
   - A urine culture will be done to r/o UTI as possible cause for preterm labor (PTL).
   - Depending on the above findings and continued contractions, she may be started on tocolytics to stop the contractions. Tocolytics that may be used include beta-adrenergic agonists (ritodrine or terbutaline), magnesium sulfate, prostaglandin inhibitors (indomethacin), or calcium channel blockers (nifedipine nicardippine).

9. **Fayola has not been drinking much for the past few days. How does dehydration relate to uterine contractions?** Dehydration may increase uterine contractility by decreasing uterine blood flow and by increasing pituitary secretion of antidiuretic hormone and oxytocin. Note: Antihistamines may cause dehydration.

10. **At the hospital triage Fayola's cervix was found to have no signs of preterm labor. She is given 500 mL of lactated ringers solution IV, the contractions stop, and after two hours of observation, they discharge her with the advice to drink more water on a regular basis. How much should she be drinking and how often?** She needs to drink at least eight 8-ounce glasses of water a day.

11. **Identify two nursing diagnoses that apply to Fayola at this time.**
    Nursing diagnoses:
    - Isolation and increased anxiety related to absence of extended family during pregnancy
    - Fluid volume deficit related to decreased intake

References

Blackburn, S. (2003). *Maternal, fetal, and neonatal physiology* (2nd ed.). St. Louis, MO: W. B. Saunders Co.

Simpson, K. R, & Creehan, P. A. (2001). *AWHONN perinatal nursing* (2nd ed.). Philadelphia: Lippincott, Williams & Wilkins.

Stan, C., Boulvain, M., Hirsbrunner-Amagbaly, P., & Pfister, R. (2003). Hydration for treatment of preterm labour. *The Cochrane Database of Systematic Reviews 2002, 2,* no. CD003096. DOI: 10.1002/14651858.CD003096.

Wheeler, L. (2002). *Nurse-midwifery handbook* (2nd ed.). Philadelphia: Lippincott, Williams & Wilkins.

Case Study 4:

Lilly

1. **List three questions that the nurse may ask that will help establish Lilly's due date.**
   - How long are your usual cycles?
   - When was your last normal menstrual period? (Lilly had not had one since before she was pregnant with her first child.)
   - When did you first begin to suspect you were pregnant? What made you suspicious?

     The nurse will be exploring subjective signs of pregnancy by trying to identify when Lilly experienced breast tenderness, nausea, and vomiting, etc.

2. **Lilly states that she felt the baby move yesterday. If this is so, how far along might Lilly be?** If this is true, then she is probably between 16 to 22 weeks. Since this is her second baby she is probably closer to 16 weeks than 22.

3. **As the pregnancy progresses, what other physical signs can be used to help confirm the due date?** Her fundal height and an early ultrasound may be helpful.

4. **Why is it important that Lilly's due date be determined during this early visit?** Due dates are only very accurate when determined early in the pregnancy. Because of her advanced maternal age (AMA), Lilly may be at increased risk for complications such as preeclampsia and gestational diabetes. If complications arise and it is determined that early delivery is necessary, it will be very important to have an accurate due date. In any case, prevention of preterm and postmature infants requires knowledge of accurate due dates for every mother.

5. **Identify two environmental factors that could possibly expose Lilly to teratogenic agents.**
   - The day care center is a source of infectious disease. It is a high-risk place for pregnant women to work.
   - Her husband may also come home from work with pesticides and fertilizers on his clothes and body that could be hazardous. He should be instructed to either shower or change before coming home, or do so immediately after he gets home and wash his clothes separately.

6. **Identify at least two other risk factors for Lilly's pregnancy?**
   - Her advanced age makes her at risk for chromosomal anomalies in this fetus.
   - She is at risk for diabetes and hypertension.
   - Closely spaced pregnancies (less than two years) may also have depleted her iron stores.
   - She is also at risk for preterm labor.

7. Lilly says that she is not ready to completely wean her 18-month-old from the breast. What advice should the nurse give her regarding this? The 18-month-old is only nursing at night and this should not pose a problem for Lilly or the baby she is carrying. Often mothers expecting their second child have a fear that they will not be as close to their first baby after the second one comes, or they could never love another child as much as they do their first one. Letting Katie take her time weaning will ease this transition for both her and the child. If Katie is still nursing after the new baby is born, this will still not cause any problems. This is called comfort nursing and is common. Depending on how much Katie is nursing after the new baby arrives, this additional physical and emotional stress can require more rest, nourishment, and psychological support for the mother. The new baby will need the colostrums for the first few days after the birth and should be nursed first. If her breasts are sore from the new pregnancy changes, Linda might try repositioning or wearing a support bra. Lilly will probably notice a decrease in her milk supply starting during the early months of the pregnancy. The nursing toddler will often complain that the milk is "all gone" or get impatient when she does not get as much milk as she is used to. Katie may also complain of a change in the taste. The toddler may find it disturbing that her place to sit (mom's lap) is disappearing as the pregnancy continues. These factors sometimes cause the older child to wean herself during the pregnancy.

8. Lilly and her husband have decided that they want their daughter present for the labor and birth. What advice should the nurse offer them regarding this decision? Their little girl will be around two years old when this baby is due. They should be sure that there is an adult at the birth who will be sensitive to her needs and will be willing to leave the birthing room any time Katie expresses, or otherwise indicates, that she does not want to be at the birth. Katie can be shown videos that show other children at birth. Her parents may have a video of Katie's birth and this could be a good start. Katie is still very young, and just as she was not that interested in the pictures in the book, she may not be interested in the birth itself. Additionally, two-year-olds can be demanding, and Lilly may find it hard to have her at the birth. The person caring for Katie needs to be sensitive to Lilly's needs to have Katie removed from the birthing room if the need arises.

9. Lilly stated that one of the children at the childcare facility where she works has been diagnosed with Fifth disease. She asks if this is dangerous to her and her baby. How should the nurse respond? Fifth disease is caused by a parvovirus. It is also known as erythema infectiosum and usually occurs in childhood. Its highest incidence is in the winter and spring. The incubation period is four to fourteen days. Initially there is usually a rash on the face that gives the appearance of being slapped. It spreads to the trunk and limbs. In the adult, the illness is usually accompanied by fever and mild arthritis along with lymphadenopathy. This is a highly communicable disease that can, if the mother were to contract it initially during pregnancy, cause severe complications to the baby, including death. About one-half of pregnant women are immune due to past exposures. The disease in an adult is mild and often without symptoms, so she would probably not know if she has had it before without testing. If Lilly is not immune, she should seriously consider not working at the center as long as there are children with the disease. When there is an outbreak in a school, about 20% of susceptible adults will contract the disease. In the fetus, the disease can cause severe anemia leading to fetal death.

10. **What test will be done to determine if Lilly is at risk for Fifth disease?** Parvovirus specific IgG and IgM test for Human B19 parvovirus will be ordered. A positive IgG and negative IgM means immunity; a positive IgG and IgM means that she has had immunity in the past and has had a recent exposure. She and the baby will probably be fine. A positive IgM and negative IgG means she was recently exposed, has or had the disease, and does not have previous immunity. This could pose serious problems for the baby.

11. **Birth centers do not offer epidurals, and many do not offer any form of medications for pain relief. Despite this, the level of satisfaction with birth center births is high, often higher than with medicated hospital births. What factors affect how satisfied a woman is with her birth experience?** The key to satisfaction is empowerment. At a woman-centered birth center, the mother is an active participant in all decisions related to her birth. Care is individualized, and even though safety is a top priority, the woman's needs and desires are considered before the needs of the staff and/or institution. Giving birth is a life experience that can have long-reaching implications on the woman throughout her lifetime. The woman who feels that "*She* is giving birth to her child" and not "being *delivered* of her child" may come away from the experience empowered and better prepared for the role of motherhood. Dependence (as when a woman is medicated and directed) enforces the role of child, whereas being treated as an individual who is making the decisions encourages the transition to parent. When a woman becomes a mother for the first time she must change the way she sees herself from her mother's child to her child's mother. Birth centers (and home births) are more likely to facilitate this transformation. Being treated with respect and provided with privacy is very important to a woman while giving birth. The birth center staff is well known to the woman and her family. Staffing is usually for the birth, not for scheduled shifts. Hospital staff is often unknown to the woman and changes by the shift as well as many times within a shift. The needs of the unit are priority. Massage and hands-on care are more likely to be a part of a birth center or home birth. "Touch and massage can convey concern, security, closeness and encouragement, and at the same time serve as a psychosocial intervention" (Chang 2002). The smaller nature of the freestanding birth center and continuity of care allow for the development of mutual trust and respect over a long period of time. All of these factors are perceived as more important to most women than pain relief alone.

References

Biancuzzo, M. (2003). *Breastfeeding the newborn: Clinical strategies for nurses* (2nd ed.). St. Louis, MO: Mosby.

Chang, Mei-Yueh, Wang, Shing-Yaw, & Chen, Chung-Hey. (2002). Effects of massage on pain and anxiety during labour: A randomized controlled trial in Taiwan. *Journal of Advanced Nursing, 38*(1).

Cartter, M. L., Farley, T. A., Rosengrens, S., Quinn, D. I., Gillespie, S. M., Gary, G. W., & Hadler, J. L. (1991). Occupational risk factors for infection with parvovirus B19 among pregnant women. *Journal of Infectious Disease, 163,* 292.

Cunningham, F. G., et al. (2001). *Williams obstetrics* (21st ed.). Norwalk, CT: Appleton & Lange.

Himenick, S. (2003, March 4). Post ecstatic birth syndrome. *Vital Signs. 13*(5).

Littleton, L., & Engebretson, J. C. (2002). *Maternal, neonatal, and women's health nursing.* Clifton Park, NY: Thomson Delmar Learning.

McCrea, B. H., & Wright, M. E. (1999). Satisfaction in childbirth and perceptions of personal control in pain relief during labour. *Journal of Advanced Nursing, 29*(4), 877–884.

Mohrbacher, N., & Stock, J. (2003). *The breastfeeding answer book* (3rd ed.). Schaumberg, IL: La Leche League International.

Riordan, J., & Auerbach, K. (2005). *Breast feeding and human lactation* (3rd ed.). Sudbury, MA: Jones and Bartlett.

Varney, H., Kriebs, J., & Gegor, C. (2004). *Varney's midwifery* (4th ed.). Boston: Jones and Bartlett.

Wheeler, L. (2002). *Nurse-Midwifery Handbook* (2nd ed.). Philadelphia: Lippincott, Williams & Wilkins.

Case Study 5: *Florence*

1. **Discuss the significance of Florence's appearance and behavior.** Her appearance may indicate that she has been hiding a pregnancy or perhaps does not have financial resources to purchase maternity clothes (although her partner seems well-dressed). In the Rastafarian belief system, the opal is thought to influence the health of the immune and reproductive systems. The acne raises questions about possible exposure to one of the teratogenic acne medications frequently prescribed for teens. As for her behaviors, as a teen she may feel embarrassed and withdrawn (related to either the pregnancy, or her obesity and acne, or all three). She may find security in being submissive to her male companion; her Jamaican culture may tend toward the quieter submissive behavior. She may fear her companion and just expect that he will insist on going with her.

2. **Discuss the significance of the companion's behaviors.** His role is not established. He could be the father, a male friend, a family member; even a stepfather (probably too young to be her father). If he is the baby's father, being from the Caribbean Islands, the age difference may not be significant, as this is common practice. Although, if they are strongly influenced by the Caribbean culture, the nurse might expect him to be less interested in the actual prenatal care. He may simply wish to protect her or to demonstrate an interest in the pregnancy; or on the other hand he may be trying to keep her from exposing an abusive relationship.

3. **Which of the following do you believe was the rationale for the nurse's behavior?**
   a. **She was establishing her authority in the clinic setting.** This is totally unnecessary and counterproductive to establishing a trusting relationship with the client. Adolescents often view authority figures with suspicion; therefore, this would be especially damaging since Florence is a teen and power plays are exactly the type of behaviors that would close communications between her and the nurse.
   b. **She was protecting Florence's privacy during the health interview.** This is one appropriate answer. All health interviews (when the client is competent and able to answer questions) need to be conducted in private. Florence needs to feel safe before she can share information with the nurse. When interacting with the adolescent, it is especially important to project a tone of

respect and provide a secure environment (physically and emotionally) in order to establish a therapeutic foundation for the client–nurse relationship. Pregnant teens, especially, have a heightened fear of exposure, both of feelings and of situation. Understanding this need for protection is essential in developing the trusting relationship. Without this trust she may withhold important history information or be afraid to express her emotional needs. In addition to insisting that Florence be seen in private, the nurse needs to reassure Florence that what she shares will be kept confidential. The nurse's behaviors must also provide a sense of security for Florence. Adolescents are especially aware of nonverbal messages. Making sure that the interview takes place in a private room with a closed door and not leaving the record sitting out where it can be picked up all demonstrate to Florence how important the nurse feels it is to keep this information confidential. *Note:* Not only is confidentiality important in order for the nurse to obtain a complete and truthful record, but in most places, it is the law.

c. **She was letting the "man" know that, although he wishes to be involved, there will be a time and a place for his involvement.** Once again, this is a power-play response and does not have any place in good nursing care.

d. **She desired to hear how Florence would answer questions, not how her companion would answer them for her.** This is also an important reason for the nurse to have Florence alone. Remember, she had observed that the registration information was being filled out by the companion without any input from Florence. It is important to elicit how Florence is feeling about her pregnancy, not how someone else is interpreting her feelings.

4. **During the interview Florence states that her last menstrual period was March 16. What is Florence's due date?** Using Naegele's Rule, the EDD is December 23. This is based on a 28-day cycle.

5. **What questions need to be answered to determine how accurate this due date is?** It must be determined if Florence has normal 28-day cycles. It is important that the nurse clarify that the last cycle was a normal cycle for Florence. Many women will have a day or two of spotting during the early pregnancy. If Florence had spotting and was not initially aware that she was pregnant, it could explain why she was so late seeking prenatal care.

6. **What are the implications of her coming so late for prenatal care?** The nurse needs to be concerned about her late entry to care. She needs to ask when Florence first suspected that she was pregnant. She may also be concerned that Florence was in denial for a period of time. How does she feel now? Finally, Florence may have been hiding her pregnancy from someone else. This, of course, would lead to concerns about her social support system.

An initial prenatal visit at one clinic may not mean "Late entry to care." She may have received care elsewhere prior to coming to this clinic. If this is so, then obtaining those records can help complete her data base. If this is her first visit, why did she wait so long before seeking prenatal care? Fear of the "system"? Ignorance of the importance of early prenatal care? Lack of transportation? Lack of financial means? These are all reasons why women do not seek early prenatal care. Sometimes prenatal care is simply not valued within the client's cultural system. If this is not the first place she sought care, then how many places has she sought care and why did she change? Sometimes clients will change caregivers due to dissatisfaction with the previous caregiver, inability to make payments, or due to relocating to a distant location. Sometimes a client is trying to hide some information from the caregiver, and when the caregiver gets too close to finding out that information, the client will flee. These may include eating disorders, use of abusive substances, or physical/emotional abuse of the pregnant woman by the partner.

7. **Nutrition is always important during pregnancy. State two reasons why the nurse needs to be especially concerned about this client's nutritional habits.** Florence is a teen, and she is obese. Even though she is overweight, she needs to understand that she needs to gain weight during the pregnancy. At 26 weeks she has gained 8 to 10 pounds. The nurse needs to review with Florence what the quality of her intake is. The nurse could ask her to do a diet history for the past 24 hours and review that at this visit or have her complete a three-day diary and review this with her at the next visit. Florence needs to understand that pregnancy is not a time for dieting.

8. **Florence is covering her acne with a heavy makeup foundation. Some acne medications are known to be teratogenic. Which ones are dangerous, and when are they the most dangerous? What advice can the nurse give Florence regarding her treatment for acne during pregnancy?** Isotretinoin (Accutane) is very teratogenic. Other formulations that are high in vitamin A may also be harmful and should be discouraged especially during the first trimester. During pregnancy the hormone changes may either help to clear the acne or make it worse. This varies from one woman to the next.

9. **What is the significance of the positive ketones in her urine?** Positive ketones in her urine indicate a lack of adequate nutritive intake and reflect the incomplete burning of fat when glucose is not available for energy. Large amounts of ketones may indicate diabetes and can be harmful to fetal central nervous system development. It is not uncommon for women to have ketones in their urine during the first trimester due to the nausea and resultant vomiting that occurs in the first 15 weeks of pregnancy.

10. **What is the implication of the positive nitrites and leukocytes esterase in the urine?** Nitrites are found when bacteria are present, providing strong suspicion of a urinary tract infection. Leukocytes indicate that the woman's body is responding to some type of infection or irritation. Sometimes, when nitrites are negative and leukocytes are positive, the cause may be contamination of vaginal discharge and not a urinary tract infection (UTI).

11. **Florence tells the nurse that her usual BP is 118-120/65-75. Describe the normal blood pressure changes in pregnancy. Does Florence's blood pressure at this initial visit fit into the normal pattern expected for this time in her pregnancy?** Blood pressure normally goes down in the second trimester due to decreased vascular resistance. By the third trimester (usually by 22 weeks) the woman's body has increased blood volume, and thus the increased vascular bed fills, returning the blood pressure to pre-pregnant levels. Elevations above pre-pregnant levels are not normal. An elevation above her pre-pregnant level at a time when blood pressure would be expected to be lower is a significant sign of possible impending pregnancy-induced hypertension and needs to be carefully monitored. In Florence's case, her early and/or pre-pregnant blood pressure is

unknown. She may have chronic hypertension, which will make her at greater risk for developing superimposed pregnancy-induced hypertension. The fact that she does not have protein in her urine at this time is reassuring, but she needs to be watched carefully.

References

Blackburn, S. (2003). *Maternal, fetal, and neonatal physiology* (2nd ed.). St. Louis, MO: W. B. Saunders Co.

Littleton, L., & Engebretson, J. C. (2002). *Maternal, neonatal, and women's health nursing.* Clifton Park, NY: Thomson Delmar Learning.

Littleton, L., & Engebretson, J. C. (2005). *Maternity nursing care.* Clifton Park, NY: Thomson Delmar Learning.

Simpson, K. R., & Creehan P. A., (2001). *AWHONN perinatal nursing* (2nd ed.). Philadelphia: Lippincott, Williams & Wilkins.

Case Study 6:   *Ruby*

1. **What is the most probable cause of her heavy irregular periods in the years just prior to menopause?** During the perimenopause, as the ovaries begin to become depleted of ova, there are fewer follicles and less estrogen and progesterone produced. Estrogen continues to build the lining of the uterus, but without progesterone withdrawal, the lining continues to grow until it outgrows the ability of the uterus to nourish it. At that time it sloughs off and causes a heavy bleed.

2. **What are the risks associated with this pregnancy?** Because of her advanced maternal age (AMA), she is at increased risk of pregnancy loss. Her age also puts her at risk for diabetes and hypertension. Her baby is at risk for congenital anomalies. In addition to the risk associated with her advanced maternal age, the fact that she is White increases the risk of her baby having cystic fibrosis.

3. **What screening tests are available to screen for congenital anomalies?**
   - Chorionic villi sampling can be done at around 10 weeks but does not screen for open neural tube defects (ONTD). *Note:* She is too late in her pregnancy for this test. This test may cause spontaneous abortion.
   - The quad/or triple test for alpha fetoprotein can screen for open neural tube defects and Down syndrome. This test is done on maternal serum, but there are many factors that increase the possibility of false results, such as obesity, uncertain or incorrect dates, multiple gestation, and diabetes.
   - Amniocentesis can be done starting at around 14 weeks gestation. This carries a risk of spontaneous abortion, infection, and placental abruption.

4. **What is Ruby's BMI?** She is five feet four inches tall and at the start of the pregnancy she was 135 pounds. This makes her BMI 22, normal. **How much weight should Ruby gain?** Ruby should gain between 25 to 35 pounds total.

5. **List at least five common signs and symptoms of menopause.**
   - Hot flashes
   - Amenorrhea
   - Fatigue

- Mood swings
- Vaginal dryness (atrophic vaginitis)
- Mental confusion and/or memory loss
- Decreased libido
- Thinning of body hair

6. **When can a woman consider herself in menopause and therefore discontinue birth control?** A woman should continue her birth control method until she has been one year without a period. Among women over 40, the rate of unplanned pregnancies is second only to the unplanned pregnancy rate among teenagers (Kasas-Annese, 1999). If a woman is taking oral contraceptives and believes she may be past the menopause and thus infertile, her follicle-stimulating hormone (FSH) and estradiol levels should be measured during the week she is off the contraceptive pill. If the level for FSH is above 30 international units per liter and her estradiol is low, it can be assumed that she is infertile. She should be tested again several weeks after she has discontinued hormonal contraceptives and she should use barrier methods during this time (Varney, 2004).

7. **What information can the nurse use to try to determine Ruby's due date?**
   - The first day of her last bleed
   - Uterine size by bimanual exam
   - Ultrasound
   - Quickening

8. **Give four possible reasons for Ruby's spotting.**
   - Ruby may be having a threatened spontaneous abortion
   - Cervicitis
   - Trauma after intercourse
   - Placenta previa

9. **Ruby's fundal height is high for the dates she reports. Name two possible reasons for this, and explain your answers.**
   - Multiple gestation is a possibility and is more common in older women.
   - She is at risk for diabetes; there is an increased risk with age.
   - If FHT had not been heard, she should also have been screened for molar pregnancy since her fundal height is high, her age is advanced, and she is also experiencing severe nausea and vomiting.
   - Ruby may be farther along in her pregnancy than would be expected from her menstrual history.

10. **What are the risks associated with hepatitis B vaccine during pregnancy.** There are none.

References

Blackburn, S. (2003). *Maternal, fetal, and neonatal physiology* (2nd ed.). St. Louis, MO: W. B. Saunders Co.

NAMS Professional Education Committee. (2004). *Menopause practice: a clinician's guide.* Cleveland, OH: North American Menopause Society.

Varney, H., Kriebs, J., & Gegor, C. (2004). *Varney's midwifery* (4th ed.). Boston: Jones and Bartlett.

Case Study 7:   *Caridad*

1. **Is there a relationship between the spotting during the first six weeks and later the intrauterine fetal death (IUFD)?** Most likely there is no relationship. Most women who have early spotting go on to have normal, uncomplicated pregnancies.

2. **Caridad is not experiencing any bleeding or cramping at this time. What is the probability that she will go into spontaneous labor soon?** Ninety percent of women who have an intrauterine fetal death will go into spontaneous abortion within three weeks.

3. **If she does not go into labor, how will the pregnancy be terminated?** If her cervix is not ripe, a prostaglandin will be used to prepare it, and then she will be induced with oxytocin.

4. **What are the risks for Caridad if she decides to wait for her body to naturally go into labor?** If her pregnancy continues beyond a month she will be at risk for developing disseminated intravascular coagulopathy (DIC). About 25% of women who maintain a dead fetus for a month or more will develop this consumptive coagulopathy.

5. **What lab work should the nurse anticipate for Caridad?** Her clotting factors will be monitored. Platelet counts, fibrin degradation products, fibrin split products, and clotting time are monitored. The D-dimer test is sometimes used as a highly sensitive and specific test for recognizing DIC in a patient. Normally, plasma does not have detectable amounts of fragment D-dimer. When present, they correlate with positive results of fibrin degradation products.

6. **What emotional and/or psychological responses should the nurse anticipate from Caridad during her labor?** The nurse can expect her to exhibit denial (she may report feeling the baby move) anger, bargaining, and depression before and during the labor.

7. **How might this experience affect Caridad in future pregnancies?** She may feel anxious and fearful when she approaches this point in future pregnancies. She may again grieve the death of this baby after the birth of another baby.

8. **How might the nurse guide Caridad's family to support her during this time?** Many times Hispanic families will try to protect the woman by limiting talk about the baby or by putting away things that were prepared for the baby. They should be encouraged to allow her to express her grief. Sometimes well-meaning families try to discount the loss with such comments as, "At least you did not lose him after he was born." The loss is very real to her regardless of the length of the pregnancy. They need to let her go through the grieving process and listen to her. They should be discouraged from putting away anything she had prepared for the baby and let her do this. Many Hispanics believe in Santeria, and that evil spirits cause illness. They may need privacy to conduct rituals to get rid of evil spirits.

9. **How likely is it that her smoking caused the fetal demise?** Smoking less than 14 cigarettes a day probably does not contribute to fetal demise. The most likely cause of the demise is cord accident. The violent movement followed by no movement is a pattern seen with cord accidents.

10. **After two weeks it is determined that Caridad needs to be induced. Her cervix is still long and closed, firm and midline. Describe how prostaglandins can be used to prepare the cervix for induction. Include nursing responsibilities**

related to safety during this procedure. She will be brought into the labor and delivery area and given prostaglandin vaginally. In some cases they may give her a prostaglandin preparation orally the night prior to try to induce her. However, the prostaglandin used orally (Cytotec) has been associated with uterine rupture and may not be a good choice with fetal demise. Prostaglandins may cause hyperstimulation leading to placenta abruption and uterine rupture, and they need careful monitoring. Depending on the type used, she will have to wait from 30 minutes to up to six hours prior to oxytocin being used to induce the contractions. Sometimes the prostaglandins themselves start contractions. She may experience nausea, vomiting, and diarrhea with the prostaglandin use. Antidiarrheal and antiemetic drugs may be used. Her vital signs will need to be monitored throughout the labor and delivery. Vaginal exams should be limited to reduce risk of infection. Pain medications may be appropriate; however, they should not be used to protect the staff from having to deal with the mother's grief. They can be used to help her deal with the physical pain of the induced birth. If they are used to cloud her cogitative senses in the hope of relieving her grief, they may do just the opposite and make it harder for her to cope with her loss. She needs emotional support. This may be in the form of a gentle touch or simply remaining at her bedside for a longer time when she is being checked. Depending on her religious preferences, she might be asked if she desires someone from her faith to be called, or the nurse can even say a prayer with her. She may wear a saint's medal or amulet for spiritual protection. The nurse should be careful when changing her gown not to lose these. These are ways of showing the mother that she is being cared for by persons who appreciate her grief and respect her need to experience it. A doula who has experience working with women delivering a dead baby would be an excellent support for her.

After the birth the mother and father should be given the opportunity to see their baby. This can be difficult since the baby has been dead for some time. Wrap the baby in a warm blanket and prepare the parents for the fact that the baby will not feel like a live baby. Encourage them to name the baby and, if they wish, to explore the baby. The nurses should refer to the baby by name. The nurses who are with her in delivery should make a point of visiting with her postpartum to allow her an opportunity to ask questions and express her grief. *Ended Beginnings* by Claudia Panuthos and Catherine Romeo provides some excellent insight into the emotional journeys parents take after the loss of a baby. The stories told by the mothers and fathers clearly demonstrate that parents, although they appear to be in a state of non-feeling during this period, are very much aware of every person around them and that these persons have a profound impact on how well the parents can process the grief for months and years afterward.

References

Panuthos, C., & Romeo, C. (1984). *Ended beginnings.* South Hadley, MA: Bergin & Garvey Publishers, Inc.

Varney, H., Kriebs, J., & Gegor, C. (2004). *Varney's midwifery* (4th ed.). Boston: Jones and Bartlett.

Case Study 8:   *Esparanza*

1. **Why was it so difficult for Esparanza to find an obstetrician who would consider doing a VBAC? Discuss the ethical dilemmas that exist when the desires and needs of the client come in conflict with those of the practitioner.** Although

VBAC in carefully selected cases is safer than repeat cesarean section, the legal ramifications if a uterine rupture were to occur have caused many obstetricians to refuse to offer this option. Other factors that discourage obstetricians from offering women this choice are that a VBAC delivery also requires that the obstetrician stay at the hospital during the active labor (whereas cesarean sections can be scheduled), and, finally, the compensation for a vaginal delivery is less than that for a cesarean section. There are many communities where this option is no longer available to women, forcing them to undergo unnecessary surgery or remain home for unassisted vaginal deliveries.

2. **What are the routine labs for this visit and why are they done at this time?** Her hemoglobin and hematocrit (H&H) will be checked. Hemodilution is greatest between 24 and 32 weeks of gestation when the woman experiences a lower hematocrit due to the rapid increase in plasma with a slower increase in RBC mass. After 32 weeks the red blood cell mass continues to increase, while the plasma volume increase occurs at a slower rate, with the result being a slight rise in H&H at the end of the third trimester. The hematocrit is checked at 36 weeks to assess maternal status near term. An anovaginal group B streptococcus (GBS) culture needs to be done. Approximately 35% of all women harbor GBS. While this seldom causes a problem for the mother, if the fetus were to become infected during the birth, the infection could become generalized, leading to critical neonatal infection and even death. When GBS is identified, the mother will be offered prophylactic antibiotics during her labor to protect the baby. The mother's urine is also checked for glucose, ketones, protein, nitrites, and leukocytes. HIV testing and testing for other STIs may be repeated at this visit.

3. **Compare and contrast VBAC and repeat cesarean section for the following: safety for both mother and baby, cost, pain, long-term effects, effects on breastfeeding, and parenting.**

Compare and Contrast

VBAC	← →	Repeat Cesarean Section
Less chance of infections; quicker recovery	**Safety for Mom**	Less chance of rupture of uterus; although risk is low if client is screened well and prostaglandins and oxytocins are not used
Baby is better able to clear excessive fluids from the lungs with a vaginal delivery	**Safety for Baby**	Safer only if VBAC resulted in uterine rupture
Less	**Cost**	More
Postpartum much less	**Pain**	Greater postpartum for extended period
Feelings of accomplishment and empowerment	**Long-term Effects**	If desired VBAC, may feel like a failure; risk for adhesions and long-range pain and complications from them
Able to breastfeed immediately	**Effects on Breastfeeding**	Often delayed; baby often gets supplements; usually decreased success rate as defined by mother
Immediate bonding and ability to hold and care for baby; earlier development of confidence on caring for baby	**Effects on Parenting**	Delayed due to pain medications for major surgery and inability to take charge of baby for an extended period

4. **Her obstetrician asks for her previous cesarean section records before he will even consider a VBAC. Why?** He will want to review the operative records to be certain that a low transverse uterine incision was made in the uterus and that there were no complications with healing after the surgery.

5. **Why are cesarean sections usually done for breech presentation?** There is no molding of the fetal head when there is a breech presentation, thus there is a greater danger of an aftercoming head being unable to pass through the pelvis. This is true especially since the smaller body parts can begin to birth with less than 10 cm dilatation (Figure 1.2 in core text). Other problems are increased risk for prolapsed cord, uterine rupture, and fractures to the infant, usually to the clavicle or humerus.

6. **When would a vaginal delivery be considered for a breech presentation?** A vaginal breech delivery may be considered when the physician is experienced in breech births and the mother is a multipara with a history of uncomplicated normal spontaneous vaginal deliveries (NSVDs); current low, but normal baby estimated fetal weight (EFW) and the presentation is a complete breech presentation. A complete breech is the position where the fetal thighs and knees are flexed.

7. **How can the baby be encouraged to move to a cephalic presentation?** There are several measures that may help. External version by the obstetrician in the hospital may change the presentation. Sometimes a tocolytic medication is used to relax the uterus while external manipulations are used to move the fetus into a more favorable presentation. This is usually done under ultrasound and with continuous fetal heart rate monitoring. If the fetus develops distress, a cesarean section is immediately done. The manipulations may cause bleeding; therefore, if the mother is Rh negative, RhoGAM needs to be given. However, after the versions these babies may reverse themselves back to breech prior to delivery. Other methods that have been used to turn a breech are having the mother try using a tilt board several times a day, moxibustion on the fifth toe, and the use of music and light to the lower pelvic area to encourage the baby to move toward them. (Moxibustion is a traditional Chinese medicine technique that involves the burning of mugwort, a small spongy herb, to facilitate healing.)

8. **What maternal/fetal conditions contribute to a baby presenting in a breech presentation?**
   ■ Uterine relaxation associated with high parity
   ■ Hydramnios
   ■ Oligohydramnios
   ■ Uterine abnormalities
   ■ Neoplasms
   ■ Contracted pelvis
   ■ Fetal anomalies
   ■ Placenta previa
   ■ CPD

9. **Compare and contrast spinal and epidural anesthesia for cesarean section.**

Compare and Contrast

Epidural	←	→	Spinal
May be used in labor if trying for a VBAC, then increased if cesarean section is needed	**Timing**		Not used for labor
Mother may feel pulling sensations but not pain	**Pain/Discomfort**		Usually does not feel anything
None	**Post Anesthesia Headache**		Possible
Often reported	**Post Anesthesia Backache**		Often reported

10. **If the baby changes to a cephalic presentation in the next two weeks but Esparanza does not go into spontaneous labor, can she be safely induced for a VBAC?** Use of prostaglandins and oxytocin for VBAC is the one factor that greatly increases risk for uterine rupture. If used, great caution and observation are needed. The obstetrician should remain within the delivery unit at all times in case an immediate cesarean section is needed.

11. **What methods can be used if any?** Induction with an attempted VBAC increases the risk for ruptured uterus. However, since the obstetrician must remain with a woman having a VBAC, he or she will often admit several women wishing VBAC who are close to their due dates and induce them at the same time.

12. **Esparanza begins to cry at the 39-week visit when she realizes that the baby has not yet changed position. She says, "I just know it's going to be terrible again. I'll never be able to breastfeed my baby postpartum; it's so painful." How should the nurse respond?** Mexican women tend to fear cesarean section and see it as life threatening to the mother (Simpson, 2001). The nurse needs to allow Esparanza to express her fears and also needs to listen to what problems she experienced last time so that she can address each one. Use open-ended statements, e.g., "Tell me about your last delivery." Esparanza may seek help from a *curanderos*, a natural healer, to try to reposition the baby.

References

Biancuzzo, M. (2003). *Breastfeeding the newborn: Clinical strategies for nurses* (2nd ed.). St Louis, MO: Mosby.

Littleton, L., & Engebretson, J. C. (2002). *Maternal, neonatal, and women's health nursing.* Clifton Park, NY: Thomson Delmar Learning.

Riordan, J., & Auerbach, K. (2005). *Breast feeding and human lactation* (3rd ed.). Sudbury, MA: Jones and Bartlett.

Simpson, K. R., & Creehan P. A. (2001). *AWHONN perinatal nursing* (2nd ed.). Philadelphia: Lippincott, Williams & Wilkins.

Tiran, D., & Mack, S. (2000). *Complementary therapies for pregnancy and childbirth* (2nd ed.). London: Baillière Tindall.

Case Study 9: *Sarah*

1. **Based on Sarah's obstetrical history, list two major concerns for this pregnancy.** A history of an LGA infant, two SAB, repeated urinary tract infections—and yeast infections, along with a baby who experienced RDS, hypoglycemia, and

early onset jaundice—is highly suspicious of gestational diabetes or even frank undiagnosed diabetes. Loss of an infant with early onset GBS is very much a concern for this pregnancy, especially with two spontaneous abortions, and repeated urinary tract infections.

2. **Review initial prenatal lab work. She is already approximately 18 weeks. What lab work is crucial for her at this time, and what can safely wait?** *Initial prenatal labs include:* PAP; DNA for chlamydia and GC; RPR or VDRL for syphilis; CBC; rubella titer; typing Rh and antibody screen; offer for AFP (triple or quad screen) screen for hepatitis B; HIV; urinalysis; and urine culture.

   In terms of the pregnancy she needs the CBC, blood typing and Rh, titers, and STI screen. She should be offered the AFP screen because it will soon be too late to do it, even if she wants it. If the urine dip is negative, further testing could wait for the next visit. However, if any of the findings are positive, then further testing needs to be done now. The rubella titer can wait since any non-immune results will only be dealt with after the baby is born. The PAP, if she has never had an abnormal PAP, can be done after the birth at the postpartum visit.

3. **What other sources might you direct this couple to for financial help?** Local community and church groups will vary with the state and city they live in.

4. **Can you predict any prenatal complications from the data previously given?** There is a very strong possibility of iron deficiency anemia.

5. **If this couple lived in your home town, what would be the options open to them for care?** Individual answers according to location.

6. **Discuss the following statement: "Not providing adequate prenatal care is much more expensive than providing it."** Caring for a preterm or injured infant or mother who has suffered from complications is far more expensive than prenatal care.

7. **If you were in a political position to change the health care system regarding maternity care, how would you change it?** Individual answers.

8. **As a student, what can you do to bring situations like this to the forefront so that individuals who have the power to change things will respond?** Nurses can write, offer to do talks at libraries and for women's groups, and so on.

9. **Discuss your professional responsibility to become involved in policy decision making regarding availability of medical care.** Nurses should become involved in their professional organizations, visit legislators, and write letters.

10. **Free clinics (those that only charge the exact cost of supplies used) or reduced-cost clinics are sometimes able to provide care at much lower fees than mainstream care facilities. One reason they can do that is volunteer professional help and another is the protection of sovereign immunity. In the past, charitable facilities were protected from lawsuits by sovereign immunity. This protection has been removed in many situations. What is the status in your area? How does having or not having sovereign immunity affect the cost of health care? Discuss the pros and cons of these legal changes.** When sovereign immunity can apply, it limits the amount that an organization can be sued for. This allows the organization and the volunteer professionals to work without paying higher malpractice

premiums. Today, malpractice premiums have driven many professionals out of the practice of maternity care. The degree to which charitable institutions can still be covered by this concept will vary according to the local/state laws.

References

Littleton, L., & Engebretson, J. C. (2002). *Maternal, neonatal, and women's health nursing.* Clifton Park, NY: Thomson Delmar Learning.

Rostant, D. M., & Cady, R. (1999). *AWHONN liability issues in perinatal nursing.* Philadelphia: Lippincott, Williams & Wilkins.

Wheeler, L. (2002). *Nurse-midwifery handbook* (2nd ed.). Philadelphia: Lippincott, Williams & Wilkins.

Case Study 10:   *Kathie*

1. **If Kathie's size equals her dates, about how many weeks pregnant do you think she is?** She has four missed periods and her fundal height, two fingers below the umbilicus, would indicate about 16 to 18 weeks.

2. **Why do you think she put off coming in for prenatal care so long?** Kathie has been in a state of denial regarding the pregnancy. She is also being unrealistic about her relationship with the baby's father and about her own limitations. Although she has been advanced in school, her ability to learn may be limited; and she is probably in special education classes. In light of her limitations, her young age, and the father of the baby's age and situation, the nurse needs to consider involving a social worker for investigation of child abuse.

3. **How important is it that her due date be established at this first visit?** This is very important. If Kathie wishes to be tested for the risk of open neural tube defects and Down syndrome, it must be done at this visit, and an accurate due date is essential for this test. In addition, the later it is in a pregnancy, the harder it is to establish an accurate due date. Ultrasounds in the second trimester may be inaccurate by several weeks in either direction and are even less accurate in the third trimester. It will be important in order to monitor Kathie regarding preterm labor and to prevent her from being post-term if she does not go into labor when she is due.

4. **In light of Kathie's advanced gestation and weight loss, how significant is her nausea and vomiting?** Kathie should be past the normal nausea and vomiting that occurs in early pregnancy related to hCG levels. Her urine dip suggests a urinary tract infection. Kathie needs to be evaluated for a kidney infection. She has a fever. She should be checked for CVAT and questioned about chills, and a urine culture and CBC need to be done. She has ketones and is losing weight. She also needs to be evaluated for hyperemesis gravidarum, and her electrolytes need to be reviewed.

5. **Which of Kathie's signs and symptoms point to a UTI? How serious are these signs and symptoms?** Symptoms that indicate probable UTI are fever and chills, pain on voiding, right lower back pain (CVAT), nausea and vomiting, positive nitrites, and leukocytes in the urine dip. These are signs of a more serious infection. They indicate that the kidneys (pyelonephritis) are involved. The physician will probably hospitalize her on IV antibiotics for several days,

especially since she is having nausea and vomiting. With vomiting, oral antibiotics may not be tolerated.

6. **What are the implications of UTI for pregnancy?** The implication for the pregnancy is that even simple bladder infections can quickly ascend to the kidneys, due to dilated and elongated ureters, and progress to pyelonephritis. In addition to the complication of the kidney infection, this also puts her at risk for preterm labor.

7. **What is the significance of the gray clinging discharge, positive whiff test, and finding of the clue cells?** This is indicative of a bacterial vaginosis infection. This can also increase her risk for a preterm labor.

8. **What are vaginal warts that turn white with ascetic acid probably from?** They are probably caused by human papilloma virus (HPV). This is a sexually transmitted condition that can increase her risk for cervical cancer. For this reason she will need more frequent PAP screens. This virus produces warts in the anogenital area. These are called condyloma acuminatum. During delivery these warts may bleed. Additionally, it is possible that the baby may pick up the virus during birth and develop the warts in her throat on the vocal cords (laryngeal papillomas). The warts can be removed during pregnancy but may recur since the virus may continue to live in the mother's system.

9. **What is the most likely reason Kathie has swollen cervical lymph glands?** She is badly in need of dental work. Given her history, she is also at risk for HIV; and swollen lymph nodes may be one of the signs of HIV infection or other generalized infection. She currently tests HIV negative.

10. **What are the implications of dental caries/infections for pregnancy?** Periodontal infections increase risk for preterm labor and birth. If she needs dental x-rays, her abdomen must be shielded. If possible it is best to avoid all x-ray exposure in pregnancy; however her dental work may require it with shielding.

11. **Discuss common misconceptions teens have about contraception.** Many teens believe that withdrawal, douching, and using various positions for intercourse will prevent pregnancy. If they do use condoms, they often also use them improperly.

12. **Make a list of topics to be discussed with Kathie as a result of this initial exam.** Pyelonephritis in pregnancy is often treated initially with hospitalization and IV antibiotics. The nurse needs to prepare her for this if the physician orders it. She will also need to be educated on the prescribed antibiotics (at home), hygiene, medications for bacterial vaginosis (BV), risk from human papilloma virus (HPV), and getting regular PAP tests. Kathie also needs to increase her intake of water. Advise Kathie not to douche.

13. **Make a list of topics to be discussed with Kathie regarding a healthy pregnancy.** Kathie needs education on pregnancy nutrition, exercise, and avoiding sexually transmitted infections (STIs). She also needs to know how to avoid getting another UTI once this one is cleared up.

14. **In light of Kathie's reading level, how will the nurse provide education?** The nurse will need to spend some extra time with Kathie discussing her needs and

checking for her understanding. She should use pamphlets written for low literacy and may try to get her involved with a small group of teens to discuss needs and questions.

References

Blackburn, S. (2003). *Maternal, fetal & neonatal physiology* (2nd ed.). St. Louis, MO: W. B. Saunders Co.

Freda, M. (2002). *Perinatal patient education.* Philadelphia: Lippincott, Williams & Wilkins.

Littleton, L., & Engebretson, J. C. (2002). *Maternal, neonatal, and women's health nursing.* Clifton Park, NY: Thomson Delmar Learning.

Morgan, G., & Hamilton, C. (2003). *Practice guidelines for obstetrics and gynecology* (2nd ed.). Philadelphia: Lippincott, Williams & Wilkins.

Simpson, K. R., & Creehan, P. A. (2001). *AWHONN perinatal nursing* (2nd ed.). Philadelphia: Lippincott, Williams & Wilkins.

Wheeler, L. (2002). *Nurse-midwifery handbook* (2nd ed.). Philadelphia: Lippincott, Williams & Wilkins.

Whitneye, N., Cataldo, C. B., and Rolfer, S. R. (2002). *Understanding normal and clinical nutrition.* Belmont, CA: Thomson/Wadsworth Publishing.

Case Study 11:   *Ruth*

1. **How many weeks gestation is Ruth at this initial visit?** Ruth is between 22 and 23 weeks gestation.

2. **Identify at least six high-risk factors that Ruth is initially presenting with.**
   - Obesity
   - Late entry into care
   - Greater than 4 pregnancies
   - Closely spaced pregnancies
   - Uncertain dates
   - Smokes one-half pack of cigarettes a day
   - Asthma
   - Previous preterm labors/birth with neonatal losses

3. **Discuss Ruth's vision changes.** Since Ruth does not have any signs of hypertension and does not complain of headaches, the most probable reason for her vision changes is a temporary change in the cornea due to the increased overall fluid retention related to the hormones of pregnancy. This is normal and will reverse after the baby is born.

4. **Native Americans have a higher risk for diabetes. Does Ruth present any indications of this problem?** Yes. Size greater than dates and fungal infection are possible signs of diabetes.

5. **During the antepartum, culture may influence what taboos and what prescriptives are needed to ensure a safe delivery (Littleton, 2001). When caring for individuals of the Native American culture the nurse should know some of the basic beliefs and behaviors that are practiced in this culture. Name four major areas where misunderstanding can occur between the non–Native American nurse and the Native American family.**
   - Many Native American children are born with Mongolian spots. Care providers often mistake these marks for child abuse.

- The quiet communication patterns that are common to the Native American population are often misinterpreted by caregivers to mean that the person is not interested. The nurse should initiate questions, offer information, and listen carefully to what is being communicated by the client to fully assess and meet the learning needs, rather than assuming that the lack of questions means that a family does not need information or resources.
- Another characteristic communication trait of the Native American is to show respect by not maintaining eye contact. This can be misinterpreted as disrespect rather than for the respect that is actually intended.
- Finally, it is important that the nurse appreciate the fact that Native American families traditionally are very family oriented and that this includes the extended families as well. Including extended family members in the care of the pregnant woman may be necessary to meet her needs (Garwick, 2000).

6. **Native Americans have higher poverty and unemployment rates than other groups of Americans. How does this affect the general health care and outcomes for Native American women?** Poverty accounts for lack of access to prenatal care, poorer nutrition, and harder physical work. Unemployment leads to depression and feelings of hopelessness. All of these factors lead to intrauterine growth retardation (IUGR) and preterm labor and birth.

7. **Aside from diabetes, what else could account for her high fundal height?**
   - Multiple gestation
   - Inaccurate dates (pregnancy further advanced)
   - Native Americans are at a higher risk for molar pregnancies; however, hearing FHT in this pregnancy would rule this out.

8. **Asthma is also more prevalent in the Native American population. Identify the risk associated with asthma in pregnancy.** Depending on the severity of the asthma, the baby's oxygen supply may be compromised. Also, if prostaglandins are given to the mother, they may cause severe asthmatic reactions. Prostaglandins are used in pregnancy to ripen the cervix and to stop postpartum hemorrhages. Examples of FDA-approved prostaglandin drugs are Cervidil, Prepidil, and Hemabate.

9. **Overall, how do the statistics on the Native American populations compare for preterm births and teen pregnancies to other populations living in the same communities?** Teen pregnancies were reported in North Carolina to be 97/1000 for Native American teens compared to 69/1000 for White teens. Prematurity associated with poverty is also much higher. Other higher risks include diabetes, hepatitis, asthma, and some STIs. The percentage of pregnant women who are Native American and smoke is also higher (N. Carolina Minority Health Facts, 1999).

10. **An ultrasound reveals that Ruth is carrying twins. Make a list of risks that are associated with multiple gestation pregnancies.** Ruth will not be able to deliver at the birth center. Although a midwife may be able to continue participating in her care, the overall management will be by an obstetrician. Some other risks include:
    - Preterm labor and birth
    - Low birth weight

- Anemia
- Preeclampsia
- Cholestasis
- Placenta previa and abruption
- Cord entanglement
- Twin-to-twin transfusion syndrome
- Acute fatty liver
- Uterine rupture
- Increased perinatal mortality
- Increased risk for fetal anomalies
- PPH (postpartum hemorrhage)

11. **Ruth goes into preterm labor at 32 weeks gestation and delivers twin boys weighing in at 3 pounds and 2 pounds 6 ounces in the hospital. Immediately following delivery of the placenta she begins to hemorrhage. Her uterus is boggy, and the obstetrician calls for carboprost tromethamine (Hemabate) stat while he does a bimanual compression. Is this an appropriate order for this client?** No. Although Hemabate is effective in controlling postpartum bleeding (Hemabate contracts the myometrium and stops bleeding), it also contracts the bronchi and smooth muscle in the gastrointestinal tract.

12. **What would have been the immediate response if the nurse had prepared the medication and the physician had given it?** Hemabate is a prostaglandin that contracts the bronchi and could have caused Ruth to have an asthmatic attack.

13. **Name two other medications that can be used for this client that will contract the uterus.** Either oxytocin (Pitocin, Syntocinon) may be used to contract the uterus postpartum to control bleeding. Methylergonovine maleate (Methergine) would be appropriate as long as the client's blood pressure is normal. It causes rapid, sustained, strong contractions. It may cause hypertension.

14. **List and explain at least four factors that placed Ruth at risk for this hemorrhage.**
    - Obesity
    - Multiple pregnancy
    - Gravida 5
    - Closely spaced pregnancies

References

Cunningham, F. G., et al. (2001). *Williams Obstetrics* (21st ed.). Norwalk, CT: Appleton & Lange.

Office for Minority Health and Center for Health Statistics. *North Carolina minority health facts: Native Americans.* (1999).

Simpson, K. R, & Creehan, P. A. (2001). *AWHONN perinatal nursing* (2nd ed.). Philadelphia: Lippincott, Williams & Wilkins.

Garwick, A. (2000). What do providers need to know about Native American culture? Recommendations from urban Indian family caregivers. *Families, Systems & Health: The Journal of Collaborative Family HealthCare, 18*(2).

Part 2: Intrapartum Case Studies

Case Study 1:　　　　　*Norma*

1. **List three questions the nurse should ask Norma at this time.**
   - Can she describe her contractions including how long they last and how far apart they are coming?
   - Is she bleeding or has her water broken; and if so, at what time? Can she estimate how much fluid there was, what was the color of the fluid, and did it have any odor (TACO)?
   - Who is with her? Does she have someone who can drive her if her contractions suddenly got stronger? The nurse should keep her on the phone long enough for several contractions to occur. By listening to the mother's voice through the contractions the nurse can estimate the intensity of the contractions.

2. **When should Norma be instructed to go to the hospital?** As long as her membranes are intact, she is not bleeding, and she is comfortable walking around at home, there is no need to rush to the hospital. When her contractions are around three to five minutes apart, lasting at least one full minute; have been doing that for about an hour; and she can no longer walk, talk, or joke throughout them, then she should consider going to the hospital. This, of course, has to be modified to come sooner if she lives a long distance or traffic could be a problem, or if she is nervous and would feel more secure being at the hospital.

3. **Norma has attended childbirth education classes. She plans to use aromatherapy, water, and massage for pain relief. How effective are these modalities in providing pain relief in labor?** These can be very effective. A restful environment allows a mother to rest and conserve her energy. Massage has been used in many forms. Both massage directly on the area that hurts or indirectly using pressure points to relieve pain can be very effective. Massage and pressure at specific sites may release endorphins, which act as natural pain inhibitors. A few drops of an essential oil in a tub of warm water can be very soothing and offer pain relief. During labor a massage with a few drops of clary sage, jasmine, lavender, nutmeg, rose, or ylang-ylang diluted in a carrier oil may give pain relief. A doula is an individual trained to provide physical and emotional labor support. They do not do medical, nursing, or midwifery procedures, nor do they offer medical advice. They can help a woman and her family understand medical events. They empower women by providing information and then support decisions that women make regarding their labor. Doulas have training and experience using these alternative modalities and can increase their effectiveness. The doula is so effective in pain management techniques that repeated studies have shown that they reduce the mother's need for epidural anesthesia by 50%.

4. **Norma has also discussed with the certified nurse midwife (CNM) the use of intermittent fetal monitoring. Discuss the pros and cons of using continuous electronic fetal monitoring in labor.** Continuous electronic monitoring in labor for the low-risk client has not been shown to improve outcomes (Feinstein, 2000). Advantages include more efficient and cost-effective management for the hospital staff (higher client to nurse ratios) and the fact that it provides a continuous record of the fetal heart rate and contractions. Disadvantages

include restriction of the mother's movement, which may interfere with fetal descent. They are also open to misinterpretation and have been shown to increase cesarean section rates without demonstrating improvement in fetal outcome. Furthermore, electronic monitoring may promote the sick role of the mother, which in turn, undermines her confidence and is disempowering. Economics has become a major influence in health care. Fetal monitors are expensive. If they were only used during high-risk labors they would not be cost-effective for hospitals to purchase and maintain.

5. **Norma has also asked that she be allowed to not have an IV in labor. Her CNM has agreed to this. Discuss the pros and cons of routine IV in labor.** Intravenous fluids in labor have been used to replace nourishment and hydration denied women in labor due to NPO policies. IVs in labor have been associated with fluid overload, hyponatremia, maternal hyperglycemia, and fetal hyperinsulinemia. When IVs are necessary (women at high risk for hemorrhage or cesarean section) only normal saline or an electrolyte solution (with or without the addition of 5% dextrose) should be used. IVs also limit maternal movement and cause increased stress, anxiety, and pain (Enkin, 2000).

6. **Furthermore, Norma has asked to be able to eat lightly and drink high-energy liquids in labor. Discuss the pros and cons of this.** This topic is strongly debated among obstetricians, midwives, anesthesiologists, nurses, and mothers. Studies conflict as to the safest and most effective ways to reduce ketones in labor and not risk aspiration should the mother need general anesthesia. Women in active labor using natural methods of pain relief tend not to desire solid foods. If left to their own desires, they usually choose foods that are easily and quickly digested such as simple carbohydrates (crackers). If a woman does eat solid foods, she would be best to take small amounts of low fat, low residue foods and avoid cold foods, which may increase gases and cause nausea and vomiting (Enkin, 2000). Narcotic analgesia may delay emptying time from the stomach, which may increase risk of aspiration if general anesthesia is needed. Some studies have shown that small amounts of oral intake of isotonic fluids do not increase risk of aspiration and do prevent ketone formation seen in starvation. These clear, high-energy drinks are better tolerated in labor and do not increase risk of vomiting. They are quickly utilized and provide the energy a woman needs for the hard work of labor (Enkin, 2000).

7. **Several hours later, Norma again calls the office to say that she feels she should go to the hospital. Her contractions are coming every three minutes and are lasting from one minute to 90 seconds. When she arrives at the hospital she is found to be 6 cm dilatated, completely effaced, and the baby is a +1 station. Her membranes are intact. The CNM gives her the option of having her membranes ruptured at this time (Figure 2.1 in core text). Discuss the pros and cons of this intervention.** Artificial rupture of the membranes (AROM) has the benefit of putting more direct pressure by the head on the cervix. Another theory is that when the uterus is less stretched, the thicker uterine wall will contract more efficiently. It is thought that this may speed the dilatation process, although this has not been well established with evidence-based studies. This additional pressure on the fetal head may increase molding and caput formation. Ruptured membranes also increase risk of pressure on the cord. If the baby were not engaged (presenting part is above zero station), rupture of

membranes would put the baby at risk for prolapsed cord. Once membranes have ruptured there is an increased risk for infection. One advantage of rupturing membranes is that it allows for the evaluation of the fluid for presence of meconium, which may indicate fetal distress and/or foul odor indicating infection. This is important if the baby's heart rate pattern raises concern.

8. **The nurse is checking the fetus and Norma's contractions intermittently. How often should they be checked?** During active labor in a low-risk labor, the fetal heart rate needs to be assessed every 30 minutes. The heart tones may be evaluated with a Feta-scope, Doppler, or external fetal monitor. It is important that the heart rate be recorded and the pattern of heart tones assessed. The nurse needs to describe the baseline and the baseline variability, and identify if any accelerations are present. If auscultation is used to listen to the fetal heart tones, the nurse can still assess long-term variability by recording 5-second rates on a graph. This takes two people. The mother or family member can assist by being the recorder, writing down the numbers as the nurse calls them out. The nurse listens and counts the heart rate for five seconds, stops for five, then listens again for five seconds throughout several contractions. Afterward, the nurse graphs them. By adding the beginning and end of contractions to the graph, the nurse can also assess the fetal heart rate for periodic patterns. These need to be described. Finally, the nurse needs to state if this is a reassuring or non-reassuring pattern.

9. **How are contractions assessed in labor?** Since Norma is having her contractions checked by intermittent monitoring, it is essential that the nurse indicate the length and duration of the contraction. The nurse must also palpate the mother's uterus to assess both the intensity of the contraction at the peak and the relaxation during the period between the contractions (tonus). The nurse needs to evaluate these factors to determine if the contractions are normal, hypertonic, or hypotonic. Adequate rest and low tone between contractions is essential for the placenta to be replenished. During the peak intensity of contractions, there is no blood flow between the maternal system and the placenta. The vessels of the uterus are compressed, preventing this exchange. If the rest period is not long enough or if the tension in the uterus remains too high at this time, a normal exchange of oxygen, nutrients, and waste products will not occur. This can occur when contractions are closer than every two minutes and lasting over 90 seconds and the uterus does not relax sufficiently (feel soft) between contractions. Deprived of this exchange, with every contraction the fetus will become further stressed and will eventually become distressed. Early signs of stress the nurse needs to be aware of are loss of accelerations of the heart rate, loss of baseline variability, and changing baseline. Soon, late decelerations are seen, and the baby is in distress. Increasing variable decelerations with overshoots at the end of the deceleration are usually a sign of cord compression.

10. **After two hours of continued strong contractions Norma is completely effaced and 10 cm dilated. Norma says she is tired, does not feel like pushing, and wants to rest prior to pushing. Discuss the pros and cons of allowing her to rest at this time.** If Norma's vital signs and the baby's heart tones are all reassuring, a period of rest can be very beneficial to both. Many women will find that they do not feel a need to push when they first reach complete dilatation.

Waiting for the normal involuntary urges to push will bring the baby down without stressing the maternal cardiovascular system or interfering with oxygenation to the fetus such as occurs with the forced pushing using the Valsalva maneuver.

References

Blackburn, S. (2003). *Maternal, fetal, and neonatal physiology* (2nd ed.). St. Louis, MO: W. B. Saunders Co.

Enkin, M., Keirse, M., Neilson, J., Crowther, C., Duley, L. E., et al. (2000). *A guide to an effective care in pregnancy and childbirth.* New York: Oxford University Press.

Feinstein, N. F., Sprague, A., & Trepanier, M. J. (2000). *Fetal heart rate auscultation.* Washington, DC: Association of Women's Health, Obstetric and Neonatal Nurses (AWHONN).

Kubli, M., Scrutton, M. J., Seed, P. T., & O'Sullivan, G. (2002). An evaluation of isotonic "sports drinks" during labor. *Anesthesia & Analgesia, 94*(2), 404–408.

Nichols, F. & Humenick, S. (2000). *Childbirth education practice, research and theory* (2nd ed.). Philadelphia: W. B. Saunders Co.

Varney, H., Kriebs, J., & Gegor, C. (2004). *Varney's midwifery* (4th ed.). Boston: Jones and Bartlett.

Walsh, L. (2001). *Midwifery community-based care during the childbearing year.* Philadelphia: W. B. Saunders Co.

Case Study 2: *Holly*

1. **What are the particular advantages for Holly in a home birth?** Holly is familiar with her surroundings. She can move about freely and has a sense of security in her own home.

2. **What coping mechanisms is Holly using to deal with the contractions? Why are these particularly good for Holly?** She is using music and dancing. Since she is blind, her hearing is extremely important to her; being able to immerse herself into music and concentrate on movement will help her avoid concentrating on pain. Movement also helps the baby move deeper into the birth canal.

3. **In general, discuss the safety of a planned home birth.** When a woman is healthy, she has had consistent prenatal care, her pregnancy has progressed normally, her home is safe and within 30 minutes of a hospital, and she is attended by qualified persons, a home birth is as safe as a routine hospital delivery (Olsen, 2003). Home birth is sometimes safer because dangerous interventions such as inductions, augmentations, and epidural and narcotic medications are not used. The mother and baby are not exposed to dangerous infectious organisms found in the hospital, and she is attended by a consistent team of professional caregivers who are able to provide undivided attention to her and her baby. All the care is individualized to meet the mother's and infant's needs. Nothing is done for the sake of efficiency of the institution. Because care providers are constant (no changing of shifts), there is less opportunity for miscommunication.

4. **Why did the midwife order a NST last week? What is the significance of a reactive NST?** A NST is a test of fetal well-being. When it is reactive, it means that the baby is able to increase his or her heart rate when more oxygen is needed, such as when he or she moves. This test is ordered when it is felt the mother may be

going past her due date or any time when the fetal well-being is in question. A reactive non-stress test usually means that the baby and placenta are doing well and will be well for about one week (barring such things as cord accidents, etc.). Due dates are only estimates, and the range of normal covers from 38 to 42 weeks. A postdate pregnancy does not always mean a post-mature fetus. Fetal assessment tests help to differentiate those pregnancies where the baby is at risk from the pregnancy going beyond the due date and those that are doing fine.

5. **What other test might she have ordered? Why?** She may have also ordered a biophysical profile (BPP). This is a more detailed test that assesses the NST and also examines the amount of amniotic fluid present, fetal tone and movement, and fetal breathing movements. The placenta may also be graded. Occasionally, an abbreviated BPP that just measures the amount of amniotic fluid, recorded as an amniotic fluid index (AFI) and an NST, are ordered. AFI decreases when pregnancy is prolonged.

6. **What are the possible consequences of a pregnancy continuing past the established date (postdate)?** Pregnancy is considered term at any point between the end of the 37th completed week and the end of the 42nd week. If a pregnancy is prolonged, the ability of the placenta to nourish and provide respiratory function for the baby may begin to decrease.

7. **What is the most important nursing action after the rupture of the membranes?** The nurse needs to check the fetal heart tones to be sure that a prolapsed cord has not occurred. This would be unlikely since this baby is already engaged.

8. **Holly continued to eat lightly and drink fluids throughout her labor. Discuss the safety of this.** Oral nourishment in labor helps sustain the mother's need for energy. Small amounts taken on a regular basis are safe. IVs and NPO became hospital standards to offset the dangers of anesthesia and procedures that increase bleeding.

9. **Describe the fetal heart pattern.** This is a reassuring pattern. Accelerations indicate a responsive baby (such as in the NST); long-term variability is also a sign of responsiveness. The baseline is wnl.

10. **How are fetal heart tones (FHTs) monitored without an electronic fetal monitor at home?** A Doppler or a fetascope can be used. These can both be used to determine long-term variability by listening throughout several contractions and rest periods and recording the 5-second readings on a graph.

11. **Holly delivers a baby boy after 45 minutes of pushing in a squatting position over an intact perineum. The baby's APGARS are 9 and 10. She then immediately puts the baby to breast. Discuss the squatting position for pushing.** Squatting allows for a larger pelvic outlet and greater ease of delivery. The main drawback is that if the mother squats for a long period of time she may become fatigued and the perineum may swell, making it more prone to tearing.

12. **What is the advantage of not cutting an episiotomy?** An episiotomy only weakens the perineum and lends itself to third- and fourth-degree tears. When a very preterm infant is to be delivered vaginally, an episiotomy will reduce pressure on the premature head. Unless the baby is in distress, it is seldom necessary to cut an episiotomy in a healthy, well-nourished woman who is delivering a full-term baby.

13. **The midwife does not cut the cord immediately, but places the baby on her mom and waits for the cord to stop pulsating. What are the advantages and disadvantages of this action?** Delayed cord clamping and cutting has been found to be associated with a higher hematocrit four hours after birth, less need for transfusion, and less intraventricular hemorrhage in preterm infants (Reynolds and Diaz-Rossello, 2004). By allowing the cord to remain intact, the infant continues to receive oxygen during the immediate period after birth. Resuscitation measures can be accomplished with the infant between the mother's legs if needed. The advantage of early cutting is that the baby can be moved to a center for easier access for interventions if needed.

14. **Aside from the benefits of the quality of the breast milk, what is the particular advantage for Holly of breastfeeding?** Holly is blind, and she will not have to worry about making formula and preparing bottles since the breast milk will always be warm and ready.

References

Littleton, L., & Engebretson, J. C. (2002). *Maternal, neonatal, and women's health nursing.* Clifton Park, NY: Thomson Delmar Learning.

Jewell, Olsen O. (2004). Home versus hospital birth. *The Cochrane Library,* 3. Chichester, UK: John Wiley & Sons, Ltd.

Rabe, H., Reynolds, G., & Diaz-Rossello, J. (2004, October). Early versus delayed umbilical cord clamping in preterm infants. *Cochrane Database System Review, 18*(4): CD003248.

Varney, H., Kriebs, J., & Gegor, C. (2004). *Varney's midwifery* (4th ed.). Boston: Jones and Bartlett.

Case Study 3: *Leticia*

1. **During a precipitous birth, what are the priorities for the baby?** Since this is an unexpected birth, there are no pre-warmed blankets for this baby. Loss of temperature occurs very quickly in a newborn (0.5 degree a minute or more) and can lead to increases in metabolism that could become life threatening. Therefore, warmth is a high priority. This includes drying the baby well and covering the head. Leticia's abdomen is warm, and placing the baby skin-to-skin on her bare abdomen is an option. Again, there are no prepared instruments; and, therefore, the nurse will need to find suction to clear the baby's mouth and nose if needed (although this baby is crying loudly and is pink) and something sterile to clamp and cut the cord. Sterility is more important than speed. The Wharton jelly will swell and stop the circulation through the cord. Therefore, the three priorities in this case with a pink, crying baby are:
   - Warmth
   - Clear airway
   - Sterile clamping and cutting of cord

2. **What are the priorities for the mother?** With a precipitous delivery, the mother is at a higher risk of birth trauma. Supporting the perineum is important to prevent tears. Coaching her to push gently will also allow the perineum to stretch slowly and not tear. This will be difficult since she is totally unprepared for the birth. This mother has been in denial and will need a lot of emotional support. She has not had prenatal care, therefore there are no records to identify if she has sexually transmitted infections (STIs), anemia, or BP problems. She is

young and overweight, both of which place her at risk for anemia and blood pressure problems. Immediate priorities at this time are:

- Prevent perineal tearing and blood loss
- Provide emotional support
- Ensure that her bladder is empty to prevent immediate postpartum hemorrhage
- Monitor for BP alterations

3. **Identify three OSHA concerns in this situation.** She is about to deliver in a regular urgent care examination room. The nurse will need to put on gloves, use eye protection, and ensure that all body fluids are cleaned up properly afterward as well as the placenta disposed of if it is not to be sent to pathology. While these are routine measures in the delivery area, they are not in a regular examination room.

4. **Is it possible for any woman to completely deny a pregnancy that goes nearly to term?** Yes. However, Leticia's trip to see her sister at this time may have been her way of seeking out someone whom she felt she could be "safe" with at this time. Corporal punishment is not uncommon in Puerto Rican families, and Leticia may have feared telling her parents.

5. **Is there any problem with Leticia receiving care as a minor without her parents present?** Until the pregnancy was discovered, Leticia's sister would have had to have a written note from their parents giving her permission to sign for Leticia's health care. However, once it was discovered that she was pregnant and this care was related to the pregnancy, Leticia could receive care on her own signature.

6. **Who is the legal guardian of the baby?** The baby's legal guardian is her mother, Leticia.

7. **What are the nursing priorities for the immediate postpartum?** These would be similar to any postpartum mother. Monitor vital signs and lochia and observe for vaginal bleeding, also monitor to be sure that the uterus remains contracted and her bladder is kept empty. Establish lactation, if this is the mother's desire, and provide emotional support. Encourage bonding with the baby.

8. **How will the nurse prepare Leticia for her discharge with her baby?** She will need extra emotional support. Her age, being single, and not having dealt with the reality of the pregnancy before birth all leave her at risk for postpartum depression. The nurse should include her sister in all instructions and give them in writing, as well as verbally, since Leticia is probably overwhelmed at this time. She should have a social worker referral for home follow-up.

9. **Leticia still denies she ever had sex. How will the father be listed on the birth certificate?** He does not have to be listed.

10. **Should the nurse suggest that Leticia breastfeed her baby?** Every mother should be encouraged to breastfeed her baby for the baby's health as well as the mother's. In this case, the baby is preterm and would definitely benefit from breast milk. Breastfeeding may also help Leticia develop a stronger bond with her baby. The nurse, however, must be sensitive to Leticia's responses when discussing breastfeeding with her and support her in her own decision if, after being informed of the advantages, Leticia wishes to bottle-feed.

References

Freda, M. (2002). *Perinatal patient education.* Philadelphia: Lippincott, Williams & Wilkins.

Rostant, D., et al. *Liability issues in perinatal nursing.* (1999). Philadelphia: Lippincott, Williams & Wilkins.

Case Study 4:   *Lydia*

1. **What are the compared risks to the mother and the infant in a cesarean section versus vaginal delivery?** The risk to the mother is much higher with a cesarean section. One study identified the risk of mortality from cesarean section to be 35.9 deaths per 100,000 deliveries with live birth outcomes from cesarean section and only 9.2 deaths per 100,000 vaginal births (ACOG News Release, July 2003). Cesarean section increases the infant risk for persistent pulmonary hypertension to four per 1000 live births. For vaginal deliveries the rate was 0.8 per 1000 live births (Levine, 2001). New studies also implicate previous cesarean sections with stillbirth in subsequent pregnancies (Smith, Pell, & Dobbie, 2003).

2. **How should the nurse approach this situation?** The nurse may start by asking her why she feels that a cesarean section is necessary and then explore her fears about vaginal delivery. It is important that the nurse also explain the advantages of waiting until labor begins to be certain that the baby is mature. The nurse could talk about the possibility of due dates being incorrect and the possibility of delivering the baby prematurely. The nurse could point out that she is a healthy woman and that labor is a natural healthy process. The nurse could discuss the fact that any time surgery is done there are also increased chances for infection or other problems and that, although cesarean section has become much safer, it is still not as safe as a normal vaginal delivery. Of course, this would have to be done through her sister.

3. **Having a cesarean section is obviously a cultural norm for Lydia. At what point do respecting culture and the risk of compromising safe care begin to conflict?** A care provider should not feel obliged to provide care that he or she believes to be unsafe or less safe. When a conflict occurs, the client can be referred to a practitioner who shares her beliefs. **How do you prioritize this dilemma?** The nurse needs to attempt to understand how different cultures place values on different types of care. Even within one culture there can be varying opinions as to what constitutes optimal care. If the nurse first tries to understand why Lydia feels the way she does, then maybe she can use this knowledge to help Lydia understand how care may differ here and why the process of vaginal birth is valued as safer for most healthy women and their babies.

4. **List at least three arguments that Lydia might use to justify her desire for a cesarean section. How should the nurse reply to each?**

   Argument: I do not wish to experience all the pain of a vaginal delivery.

   Response: Cesarean section is a major surgery, and the pain afterward lasts much longer than the pain from a vaginal delivery.

   Argument: A cesarean section is safer for my baby.

Response: Actually, unless there is a problem, a vaginal delivery prepares your baby better for the transition to life outside of the uterus than a cesarean section does. The stimulation of moving through the birth canal is beneficial to the baby. During the 2nd stage of labor there is an increase of catecholamines in the fetus 5 times greater than in the mother. These also help clear the fetal lungs.

Argument: I will probably have a cesarean section anyway so why go through labor?

Response: With cesarean sections at over 50% and higher in many areas, there is a 1 out of 2 chance that anyone will have a cesarean section. If she wants an operative delivery, her chances are even higher.

5. **What are the possibilities that, if Lydia were to go into labor, she would still need a cesarean section?** She is very likely to have a cesarean section.

6. **Are they increased over another woman who does not desire a cesarean section?** Her chances of failure to progress (FTP) are increased. The mind is a powerful component in a woman's labor. Gayle Peterson's work investigated how much of an influence a woman's mind can have over her labor. She used the phrase "As a woman lives so shall she labor" (Peterson, 1981) to explain why in some cases there is no physical reason why a labor will not continue, but the woman herself has a strong history of avoiding stressful situations and just allows her body to stop whatever it is that she will not face.

7. **Lydia, against her wishes, is given an appointment to come back at 39 weeks. She tells her sister in Spanish, "This country is so backward. I would never have to tolerate this pregnancy this long back home." She then begins to cry. The sister explains this to the nurse. How should the nurse reply?** *Reply:* Pregnancy lasts for 10 four-week months or forty weeks. It is safer for the mother and the baby to complete as much of that time as possible without interference. Although elective cesarean section is becoming more common, clinical trials have not been completed that validate this liberal use (Rayburn and Zhang, 2002). Induction is not even advised for suspected macrosomia (Irion and Boulvain, 2003). One reason for this is that due dates may be incorrect and the baby may be induced early.

8. **The nurse would like to offer Lydia some classes on labor preparation. How might this sensitive topic be approached?** The nurse might suggest that classes may be helpful in giving Lydia tools to deal with the postpartum discomfort, as well as help her through the last few days of pregnancy.

9. **At the 39-week visit, Lydia is obviously angry and again, through her sister, insists on ending this pregnancy tonight with a cesarean section. "Why do they make me suffer so?" she asks her sister who interprets for the nurse. It is obvious that Lydia is used to getting her own way. Her BP is 148/76; FHTs at the left lower quadrant (LLQ) are in the 150s. She has lost two pounds in the past week and states that the baby is not moving as much as before. The obstetrician orders an NST that is reactive. Her Bishop score is 8. He also offers to induce her with an epidural if she wishes. Explain the BP elevation and weight loss. She accepts the induction if "I will not feel any pain."** Stress will elevate the systolic BP without really causing much change to the diastolic reading. A weight loss of several pounds is common just prior to labor starting. Also she may have been so upset that she was not eating well.

10. **What is a Bishop score?** The Bishop score is an assessment of the cervix that determines if it is inducible. A score of 9 or greater indicates a good possibility that an induction will result in effective active labor.

Score	Dilatation	Effacement	Station	Cervical Consistency	Cervical Position
0	Closed	0–30	−3	Firm	Posterior
1	1–2	40–50	−2	Medium	Midposition
2	3–4	60–70	−1.0	Soft	Anterior
3	≥5	≥80	+1, +2	—	—

11. **Six hours into the labor with the epidural, Lydia has only dilated to 4 cm, is 100% effaced, and at zero station. She delivers via a cesarean section for failure to progress (FTP). Discuss this outcome.** Lydia may not have progressed for many reasons. Her Bishop score was good, but still less than 9. Due to the epidural causing her to be immobile and relaxing the pelvic muscles, the baby may have failed to rotate and descend (Howell, 2003). Or her failure to progress may be a result of her strong desire for a cesarean section. The mind is a very strong influence and may have been the prime factor that did not allow her labor to progress to vaginal delivery. If Lydia was really set against a vaginal delivery, there was a good possibility that she would not deliver vaginally.

References

ACOG News Release. (2003). Weighing the pros and cons of cesarean delivery. http://www.acog.org/from_home/publicatons/press_releases/nr07-31-03-3.cfm.

Blackburn, S. (2003). *Maternal, fetal, and neonatal physiology* (2nd ed.). St. Louis, MO: W. B. Saunders Co.

Cunningham, F. G., Gant, N., Leveno, K., Gilstrap, L., Hauth, J. C., & Wenstrom, K. (2001). *Williams Obstetrics* (21st ed.). Norwalk, CT: Appleton & Lange.

Howell, C. J. (2003). Epidural verses non-epidural analgesia for pain relief in labor. *The Cochrane Library,* 3. Oxford: Update Software.

Irion, O., & Boulvain, M. (2003). Induction of labour for suspected fetal macrosomia. *The Cochrane Library,* 3. Oxford: Update Software.

Levine, E. M., et al. (2001, March). Mode of delivery and risk of respiratory diseases in newborns. *Obstetrics & Gynecology, 97*(3), 439–442.

Peterson, G. (1981). *Birthing normally.* Berkeley, CA: Mindbody Press.

Rayburn, W. F., & Zhang, J. (2002). Rising rates of labor induction: present concerns and future strategies. *Obstetrics & Gynecology, 100*(1), 164–167.

Smith, G. C., Pell, J. P., & Dobbie, R. (2003). Caesarean section and risk of unexplained stillbirth in subsequent pregnancy. *Lancet, 362*(9398), 1779–1784.

Case Study 5:   *Kathleen*

1. **What questions does the nurse need to ask Kathleen to assess her contractions?** Have her describe the character of the contractions. Has she been timing them and, if so, are they getting closer, longer, and stronger? When she changes her activity do they decrease, go away, or get stronger?

2. **How do true labor contractions feel to the woman, as opposed to Braxton Hicks contractions?** Braxton Hicks will tend to ball up in front while true labor

will usually radiate from the back to the front. Braxton Hicks may go away with activity change.

3. **What is the significance of the FHT?** Accelerations are a reassuring sign of fetal well-being; however, hers are heard best just above the level of the umbilicus, which should raise strong suspicion of a breech presentation. Leopold's maneuvers should be used to try to determine the fetal presentation. An ultrasound should be used to confirm the presentation.

4. **What further information is needed from the vaginal exam (VE) to assess her condition?**
    - What is the presenting part? If it is breech, a transport to the hospital is necessary.
    - Is it engaged?
    - Are the membranes ruptured?
    - What is the character of the vaginal discharge?
    - Is a show present?

5. **What is the significance of the vaginal discharge?** Vaginal discharge may be ruptured membranes, bloody show, vaginal infection, or normal leucorrhoea, which is increased with pregnancy.

6. **How will the nurse check to see if the membranes have ruptured?** A sterile vaginal exam should be done; and the fluid can be checked by either nitrazine test, which will turn the tape blue if it is amniotic fluid, or by putting some fluid on a slide, letting it dry, and looking at it under a microscope. Amniotic fluid will look like a fern pattern on the slide.

7. **If the baby were not engaged, would it pose a problem at this stage of labor?** This mother is a multigravida, and often because of lax abdominal muscles, the baby is not directed effectively into the pelvis and the baby does not engage until labor has progressed further. However, there is concern that this baby may be breech. That is a major concern and must be ruled out before she can be allowed to continue to birth at the birthing center. If her membranes have ruptured and the baby is not engaged, she would also be at risk for prolapse of the umbilical cord. If the baby is in a breech presentation, this risk for cord prolapse is increased.

8. **What is the significance of the fact that she is deaf?** Deaf clients may respond in ways that are different from hearing clients. They may react as if they feel that they are dependent and need to be cared for, or they may act more independently and may reject approaches by the care provider, feeling that the care provider cannot understand how they feel or think since "I am deaf and you are not."

9. **What is the best way for the nurse to communicate with Kathleen since she is deaf?** The nurse should be careful about abruptly shifting topics. It is difficult for deaf clients to have a topic changed without some kind of transition or period of break (silence) that will signal the end of one conversation and start of another. Kathleen's husband is present and can communicate with her; however, she should be offered a deaf interpreter if she knows sign language. Not all women wish to have their husbands present for the labor and delivery, and she has the right to have someone else there for communication if this is her

desire. Kathleen may read lips and, if so, the nurse has to be sure to face Kathleen at all times when speaking and to speak at a normal pace. Kathleen may also prefer to have important things written down.

10. **What is the significance if Kathleen's membranes are ruptured and meconium is present?** If the baby was in a breech presentation, the meconium would be an expected finding due to pressure on the presenting buttocks. However, whatever the cause of the meconium in the fluid, the fact that it is there poses risk for aspiration by the baby. The degree of meconium is important to note. Light-stained meconium usually does not pose a risk, while heavy-particulate meconium (sometimes called pea soup meconium) can be dangerous and even life threatening to the baby if aspirated. This is called meconium aspiration syndrome (MAS).

11. **If Kathleen is in active labor, will she be allowed to deliver in the freestanding birth center?** Although as a Christian Scientist she may feel more comfortable at the birth center, there are two concerns presented:
    - If the baby is breech, she should not be delivered outside of a hospital setting.
    - If meconium is present this early in the labor and it is any more than light staining, she should be transported to a hospital while it is still early and easy to do so.

References

Newbold II, H. (1979, March). Social work with the deaf: a model. *Social Work, 24*(2), 154.

Caissie, R. (2000). Conversation topic shifting and its effect on communication breakdowns for individuals with hearing loss. *Volta Review, 102*(2).

Herring, R., & Hock, I. (2000, February). Communicating with patients who have hearing loss. *NJ Medical, 97*(2), 45–49.

Iezzoni, L. I., O'Day, B. L., Killeen, M., & Harket, H. (2004, March). Communicating about health care: Observations from persons who are deaf or hard of hearing. *Ann Intern Med., 140*(5), 356–362.

Case Study 6:   *Cassandra*

1. **Is the fact that she is still a negative 2 station significant?** Since she is a multigravida there is not as much concern as there would be with a primigravida. Due to decreased abdominal muscle tone, it is not uncommon for multiparas to keep their babies higher until later in the labor and then have a fairly rapid descent.

2. **Assess the following data: FHT 150s, no accelerations, minimal variability, no decelerations, baby is moving during rest periods between contractions.** This is a change from her earlier findings. The baseline is increasing and this may be an early warning sign of possible stress or developing infection (increased maternal metabolic rate often seen just prior to temperature elevation). In this case the maternal temperature is elevating. This may be a result of the epidural, which is not an unusual side effect. Loss of accelerations and decrease in variability are signs of increasing stress; however, the baby is probably not in true distress since there are no decelerations noted at this time. Since the baby is moving and there are no accelerations, this could be interpreted as a non-reactive pattern. This is a non-reassuring sign. *Assessment:* FHTs guarded,

indicating signs of increasing stress, no impending signs of hypoxia at this time. The fetus may benefit by a change in the maternal position at this time. Increasing the IV flow (without Pitocin) sometimes improves the FHT pattern.

3. **What is the rationale for the ampicillin?** The mother has positive GBS, and this is prophylactic to protect the baby. The Centers for Disease Control and Prevention (CDC) recommends prophylactic treatment to protect the baby, in labor, for all women who are GBS positive during the pregnancy.

4. **Cassandra had desired a natural home birth with no pain medications. What factors led up to her requesting an epidural?** Cassandra is exhausted and disappointed about the transfer. The Pitocin causes harder and closer contractions, which are more painful to deal with. She is in an unfamiliar environment, surrounded by strangers and machines, and unable to walk around. All of these things make the contractions more difficult to cope with.

5. **Two hours later she is 100% effaced and 10 cm dilated (complete, complete). With encouragement she pushed for two hours and managed to push the head out. Immediately the head turtles. What does the term *turtle* mean?** The baby's shoulders have impacted over the symphysis pubis, and the baby is now unable to descend. This is called shoulder dystocia and can be life threatening. The baby's head will begin to turn dark blue to black as circulation becomes trapped in the baby's head. Position of the head and neck and compression of the baby's abdomen and chest all make it impossible for venous return to occur. This excessive intravascular pressure deprives the baby of oxygen and may even be accompanied by intracranial hemorrhages. Brain damage and death may occur if the baby is not delivered quickly. Time is called out loud to keep the providers aware of how long the situation has existed. After only a few minutes, anoxia and excessive intravascular pressure may cause irreparable brain damage or even death.

6. **What are the causes of shoulder dystocia (Figure 2.3 in core text)?** Women who are five feet tall and under are at a greater risk. Just the fact that her labor slowed is often a sign that this labor will not progress. Any labor that needs augmentation should be carefully monitored. Other causes are short umbilical cord, abdominal or thoracic enlargement of infants (often seen in infants of diabetic mothers), locked or conjoined twins, uterine constriction ring, and true shoulder dystocia.

7. **What position should the nurse assist Cassandra into in order to assist the obstetrician in the delivery of the shoulders? (List two possible positions that may be helpful at this time and explain why they can help.)** The most common position used is McRobert's maneuver. In this position the mother's legs are bent and the knees are forced back against her shoulders with the knees out to the sides. This mimics a squatting position but keeps her in a position where the person doing the delivery can insert her or his hands into the pelvis on the baby's chest and back and assist in rotating the baby under the pubic bone. This is called the corkscrew maneuver. A second position that may work by itself is the hands-and-knees position (Gaskin maneuver). This uses gravity to help free the shoulders.

8. **Distinguish between supra pubic pressure and fundal pressure (Figure 2.4 in core text).** Fundal pressure is controversial and is pressure applied at the fundus of the uterus downward, pushing the baby out. It is used most often when

a mother cannot push well with an epidural. If the mother and/or baby are not in danger, the better policy would be (1) not to top off epidurals close to pushing time and (2) if the epidural is interfering with the maternal ability to push, wait for it to wear off. Fundal pressure may result in a ruptured uterus, placenta abruptions, and/or excessive fetal to maternal transfusion. Super pubic pressure is downward pressure just above the symphysis pubis used to dislodge a trapped shoulder.

9. **Which one will help to deliver the shoulders and why?** Fundal pressure during shoulder dystocia may further impact the shoulder, making it harder to free the baby. Supra pubic pressure is used to dislodge a fetal shoulder and push it under the pubic bone so that the baby can be rotated and free the shoulder.

10. **What measures should the nurse be taking to prepare for immediate care of this newborn?** This baby will probably need full resuscitation. A neonatal team should be present at the delivery and all resuscitation equipment ready to use.

11. **What possible injuries might this baby sustain as a result of this delivery?** This baby may develop brain damage, from anoxia and intracranial hemorrhages, and even death. In an effort to free the shoulders, he may also suffer strain on the brachial plexus and/or fractured clavicle.

12. **What injuries might the mother sustain?** The mother may have increased lacerations, rupture of the uterus, and/or hemorrhage. Traumatic deliveries also increase risk for amniotic fluid emboli.

References

Center for Disease Control and Prevention. http://www.cdc.gov.

Littleton, L., & Engebretson, J. C. (2002). *Maternal, neonatal, and women's health nursing.* Clifton Park, NY: Thomson Delmar Learning.

Varney, H., Kriebs, J., & Gegor, C. (2004). *Varney's midwifery* (4th ed.). Boston: Jones and Bartlett.

Case Study 7:   *Mimi*

1. **Shortly after Mimi is admitted to the labor suite she starts to push. The nurse checks her and finds that she is 7 cm and still at −1 station. What problems can result from Mimi's pushing at this time in the labor?** If Mimi pushes prior to complete dilation, she may cause the cervix to swell and close. It is even possible that pushing can cause tears to the cervix with the possibility of tearing further up the uterus.

2. **How can the nurse help Mimi stop pushing at this time?** The nurse should direct Mimi to blow gently when she feels the urge to push. Blowing may cause Mimi to hyperventilate. To avoid this, the nurse should have her cup her hands and breathe into them. The nurse also needs to explain to Mimi the reason why she should not push at this time. She may position Mimi on her side. This may reduce some of Mimi's urge to push prematurely.

3. **What is the significance of the meconium in the fluid?** Meconium in the fluid may indicate that the baby is post-mature and/or in distress.

4. **What special preparations will the nurse make to care for this infant immediately after birth?** Adequate suction needs to be ready for the birth. When moderate amounts of meconium are identified in the amniotic fluid, the standard of care has been to do deep suctioning of the infant prior to the shoulders being born. This was thought to reduce the amount of meconium the baby may aspirate. However, at least one recent study has questioned this procedure (Vain, 2004). The nurse also needs to make preparations for resuscitation. In many hospitals this means that a special team be present for the delivery. Usually this team consists of a neonatal nurse practitioner or a special resuscitation team.

5. **The baby's head is in anterior asynclitism. What factors may account for this position?** This is Mimi's third pregnancy in three years. Her abdominal muscles are lax and are allowing the uterus and baby to fall forward.

6. **The head engages. What problems can occur if the baby remains in a persistent asynclitic presentation?** Asynclitic presentation means that the fetal head is entering the pelvis in lateral flexion (tilted) to one side. This puts one parietal bone deeper into the pelvis than the other. Usually, it is the posterior parietal bone that enters first. Once the anterior parietal eminence descends, the fetal head is once again synclitic. While an asynclitic engagement allows for passage of a larger head through the inlet than would otherwise be able to pass, if the infant stays asycnlitic deep in the pelvis, it may prevent normal internal rotation.

7. **What can be done to help direct the fetal head into the pelvis and convert the head to a synclitic presentation?** The nurse can assist the mother into a supported-squat position. The mother will lean backward against a partner, who holds her under the arms and takes all her weight. Between the contractions she will stand. This position lengthens her trunk and allows more room for an asynclitic baby to rotate.

8. **Three hours after admission the nurse notes that the baby's head is beginning to form a large caput. Fetal heart tones are noted to decrease to 110 bpm around the height of the contractions and return to the baseline of 130s, just prior to the end of the contractions. What is the significance of these observations?** A large caput will form when there is pressure from above and resistance from below. This is often seen when there is inadequate room for the head to descend. The nurse needs to be aware that cephalopelvic disproportion (CPD) may be occurring. She needs to monitor the fetal descent carefully. The fetal heart rate pattern is that of early deceleration. This is a normal fetal heart pattern response to pressure on the head and on the vagal nerve.

9. **Bloody show is increasing and Mimi has an increased urge to push. The nurse checks her and finds that she has an anterior cervical lip. What might the nurse do to help reduce the lip and prepare Mini to deliver?** The nurse needs to position Mimi to keep pressure off the anterior cervix. It is possible that the nurse or physician can gently push the cervix over the baby's head as she pushes gently with a contraction.

10. **After the lip is reduced, the baby begins to descend rapidly. The infant is crowning and the heart tones fall to 90s. The physician is preparing to deliver the head in the next few contractions. Identify two nursing actions that are appropriate at this time.** The nurse needs to put an oxygen mask on the mother

set at 10 to 12 liters a minute. The IV flow rate also needs to be increased if no Pitocin is present in the IV.

References

Cunningham, F. G., Gant, N., Leveno, K., Gilstrap, L., Hauth, J. C., & Wenstrom, K. (2001). *Williams Obstetrics* (21st ed.). Norwalk, CT: Appleton & Lange.

Nichols, F., & Humenick, S. (2000). *Childbirth education practice, research, and theory* (2nd ed.). Philadelphia: W. B. Saunders Co.

Vain, N. E., Szyld, E. G., Prudent, L. M., Wiswell, T. E., Aguilar, A. M., & Vivas, N. I. (2004). Oropharyngeal and nasopharyngeal suctioning of meconium-stained neonates before delivery of their shoulders: Multicentre, randomised controlled trial. *Lancet, 364*(9434), 597–602.

Case Study 8:   *Danielle*

1. **Is there any significance to the fact that Danielle is 41 years old?** Older primigravidas are more likely than younger mothers to have long prodromal labors. She would have been well advised of this ahead of time so that she does not come to the hospital too early. Advanced maternal age has been associated with increased risk of hypertension and diabetes and increased fetal loss. Perinatal mortality, intrauterine fetal death, and neonatal death increase with age of mother (Jacobsson, Ladfors, and Milsom, 2004). Even when the mother is in excellent health, older primigravidas also are more often given cesarean sections due to the belief that these are premium babies, meaning that her ability to conceive again is less than for a younger woman and this could be her only baby. Along with this belief, many obstetricians have an innate distrust of birth, considering all births as risky. Cesarean section increases risk for the mother and baby in this pregnancy and in future pregnancies (CIMS, 2003). Persistent pulmonary hypertension for babies born via elective cesarean section without labors occurs five times more often than those delivered vaginally (Levine, 2001). Infection rates are also higher following cesarean sections. Contrary to these and other evidence-based studies that clearly demonstrate vaginal birth as safer than cesarean section (Scott, 2002), older women are more likely to be delivered surgically "to ensure healthier babies."

2. **Is there any significance to the fact that this is her first pregnancy?** Primigravidas (women pregnant for the first time) will usually experience the baby moving deeper into the pelvis about two weeks prior to the baby's birth. This is called lightening. Primigravidas generally have stronger abdominal muscles, and these strong muscles direct the baby's head into the pelvis better than the already stretched muscles of a multigravida. When lightening occurs, the baby's head enters into the pelvic inlet and usually the leading presenting part is at the ischial spines. When this occurs, the baby is said to be at zero station. The fact that Danielle was still at a −3 station (approximately three centimeters above the ischial spines) may be a warning sign that the baby may have problems entering the pelvis and be more likely to experience cephlopelvic disproportion (CPD).

3. **Discuss Danielle's dreams.** Pregnant women commonly have dreams about birth and babies. Dreams often do the emotional work that a person's conscious self does not feel prepared to deal with. Toward the end of pregnancy, as

a woman prepares for the separation of her baby from her body, she may dream of misplacing the baby or of being trapped in a small place (Frye, 1995).

4. **What is the significance of the +2 pitting edema in her ankles?** Some dependent edema is normal in pregnancy during the third trimester. It can be considered a positive reflection of the increased circulating blood volume. This increased circulating fluid volume and pressure of the pelvic veins impeding return circulation make this a common finding. Plus two pitting edema is a little more than expected; however, since she is spending hours standing on her feet, it is probably understandable. This is especially true since she does not have any other edema; it is not present when she gets up in the morning, and it goes away after she gets off her feet and lies down.

5. **What advantages or disadvantages are there to cesarean section following labor as opposed to scheduled cesarean section?** The advantages are that the labor releases catecholamines in the baby's systems that help to clear the fluid from the baby's lungs after birth. Catecholamines stimulate the secretion of surfactant into the alveolar space. In the second stage, the levels are actually five times higher in the infant than in the mother. These increased levels help the baby to clear his or her lungs of the fluid that is naturally there prior to birth. If a woman is delivered without labor, as in a scheduled cesarean section, the baby will find it more difficult to clear this fluid (Levine, 2001). The disadvantage is increased maternal fatigue from the hours of labor, and if invasive procedures were a part of the labor (as they were in this case—AROM and internal monitoring), there is increased risk of infection.

6. **List the indications and risk of artificial rupture of membranes (AROM).** AROM is done to examine the amniotic fluid for signs of meconium to determine possible fetal distress, to speed labor, and to insert internal fetal and uterine monitoring devices. Risks of AROM are increased risk of infection, possible injury to the baby related to increased pressure on the baby, and increased risk of cord prolapse if the baby is not engaged. AROM is also associated with increased cesarean section rates (Fraser, Turcot, Krauss, and Brisson-Carrol, 2003).

7. **Why do you think a cesarean section was done?** Danielle is a primigravida in labor with a baby at a −3 station. Most primigravidas will start labor with the baby engaged. This mother was just 38 weeks; therefore, there is some possibility that lightening has just not had the chance to occur and would have any day. The mother's description of her labor prior to hospital admission leaves some doubt that it was active labor and perhaps she was experiencing Braxton Hicks contractions and not labor. If the baby's heart tones were reassuring and her membranes were intact, she would have been better advised to go home and wait for labor to get stronger on its own. Augmenting a labor that is not well-established and artificial rupture of membranes at this early stage increase the chances of failure to progress and cesarean section. If the gap junctions (the cell-to-cell communications system within the myometrium that develops at term and allows coordinated labor contractions) and oxytocin receptors have not been established prior to induction and/or augmentation, labor will not progress. Another concern is that the membranes were artificially ruptured at a −3 station. This increases risk of prolapsed cord. Other factors in this cesarean section could be that it was Friday afternoon and the mother already had an epidural anesthesia. With the changing economic and political influences in maternity

care, the tendency to do cesarean sections earlier is becoming more common (Hodges, 2004).

8. What is the difference between Pitocin induction and Pitocin augmentation? Induction refers to labors that have not started on their own and are being initiated with Pitocin. Augmentation is when labor has started but is not effective and is being enhanced with Pitocin.

9. Analyze the information given regarding the fetal heart tones. The initial heart tones indicated good variability and reassuring patterns of accelerations. As the labor progressed, and after the AROM, there was evidence of fetal stress indicated by the decreases in variability and variable decelerations (a sign of possible cord compression or prolapse). Cord compression/prolapse is the best explanation since a change in the maternal position stopped the variable decelerations.

10. Why did the variable decelerations stop after the client was positioned on her right side? Changing the maternal position relieves pressure on the cord. Rupturing membranes prior to engagement increases risk of prolapsed cord. The cord can slip forward of the presenting part and be compressed as gravity and the contractions bring the baby down. More likely, the cord was being compressed between the pelvis and the baby's head since the baby only showed signs of stress (increasing variable decelerations) that were relieved by placing the mother on her side. This probably would not have occurred if the membranes had still been intact. **What other positions might have been used?** She may have been put in a knee-chest position to relieve the pressure.

11. What effect might having an epidural have had on this labor and the cesarean section outcome? When a woman is in early labor and has an epidural, she is at the disadvantage of not being able to walk around. Since this baby was high in the pelvis and initially the membranes were intact, she might have benefited by an upright position and activities that gently rocked the pelvis to help the baby descend (walking up and down stairs, pelvic rocking, lunges, sitting on a birthing ball, or swaying). When women feel their contractions, they naturally will change their positions to ones that relieve pressure. These same positions often assist the baby to move deeper into the pelvis. Women in bed with an epidural do not feel the contractions and pressure and therefore cannot react to these signals. Furthermore, epidural anesthesia relaxes the pelvic muscles and may interfere with fetal descent. In first-time mothers, epidurals have been shown to increase the rate of cesarean section (Howell, 2003).

12. What else might have been done to help the baby descend and labor progress? There are several acupressure points that can enhance contractions and descent. The first of these is called Kidney 1 in Chinese medicine (Yongquan), and it is used to help descend the baby and relax the perineum. Apply pressure by using your thumb and press firmly at the center of the ball of the foot. Enhance contractions by stimulating the point LI 4 (Hoku). This may be done by pinching the skin at the web of the thumb next to the metacarpal of the index finger. Ice may also be applied to this point to stimulate it.

References

ACOG. Evaluation of cesarean delivery. (2000). Washington, DC: ACOG.

American Academy of Pediatrics. (2005, February). Policy statement: Breastfeeding and the use of human milk. *Pediatrics 115*(2), 496–506.

Blackburn, S. (2003). *Maternal, fetal, and neonatal physiology* (2nd ed.). St. Louis, MO: W. B. Saunders Co.

CIMS Coalition for Improving Maternity Services. (2003). *The risks of cesarean section to mother and baby: a CIMS fact sheet.* http://www.motherfriendly.org/Downloads/csec-fact-sheet.pdf.

Fraser, W., Turcot, L., Krauss, I., & Brisson-Carrol, G. (2003). Amniotomy for shortening sponta-neous labour. *The Cochrane Library,* 2. Oxford: Update Software.

Frye, A. (1995). Holistic midwifery care during pregnancy, 1. Portland, OR: Labrys Press.

Hodgess, S., & Goer, H. (2004). Effects of hospital economics on maternity care. *Citizens for Midwifery News.*

Howell, C. J. (2003). Epidural verses non-epidural analgesia for pain relief in labor. *The Cochrane Library,* 3. Oxford: Update Software.

Jacobsson, B., Ladfors, L., & Milsom, I. (2004, October). Advanced maternal age and adverse perinatal outcome. *Obstetrics & Gynecology, 104*(4), 727–733.

Levine, E. M., Ghai, V., Barton, J. J., & Strom, C. M. (2001). Mode of delivery and risk of respi-ratory diseases of newborns. *Obstetrics & Gynecology, 97*(3), 439–442.

Littleton, L., and Engebretson, J. C. (2002). *Maternal, neonatal, and women's health nursing,* Clifton Park, NY: Thomson Delmar Learning.

Lydon-Rochelle, M., Holt, V. L., Easterling, T. R., & Martin, D. P. (2001). First birth cesarean and placenta abruption or previa at second birth. *Obstetrics & Gynecology, 97(5PT1),* 765–769.

Scott, J. R. (2002). Putting elective cesarean into perspective. *Obstetrics & Gynecology, 99,* 967–968.

Waters, B., & Raisler, J. (2003). Ice massage for the reduction of labor pain. *Journal of Midwifery and Women's Health.* New York: Elsevier.

Young, A. (2002). Acupuncture pain relief for the midwife. *Acupuncture Newsletter,* Miami.

Case Study 9:   *Josie*

1. **The midwife calls the nurse to assist in positioning Josie. What position will they place her in?** They will either place her in a knee-chest or Trendelenberg position with the hips elevated and head low. This will facilitate getting the weight of the baby's head off the cord.

2. **What are the risks associated with prolapsed cord?** When the cord presents in front of the baby, the weight of the baby puts pressure on the cord, reducing or stopping the blood flow. If not corrected immediately, the baby will die.

3. **What factors contributed to the cord prolapsing?** Prolapsed cord occurs when:
   ■ There is rupture of the membranes and the baby is not engaged.
   ■ The baby is not in a cephalic presentation.
   ■ There is rupture of membranes in a preterm baby.
   ■ There is a long cord.
   ■ The placenta is low lying.
   ■ There is a multiple gestation.

   A prolapsed cord may be obvious and visible outside of the vagina or occult and only detected by checking the fetal heart tones.

4. **While the midwife does a vaginal exam, the nurse checks the fetal heart tones. What patterns might the nurse expect to hear?** If there is only slight intermit-tent pressure on the cord, as occasionally occurs in labor when the baby de-scends, the pattern is one of variable decelerations. Continued pressure on the cord will cause a fetal bradycardia.

5. **What other immediate actions are needed at this time?**
    - The midwife will need to keep her hand in the birth canal to hold the baby's head off the cord.
    - Determine if the mother is completely dilated and if a vaginal delivery would be more expedient.
    - The nurse will have to call for help, call for an ambulance, and alert the hospital and backup physician of the transport and the prolapsed cord.
    - The mother should be given oxygen by a well-fitting face mask at 10 to 12 liters/minute.
    - A copy of the mother's chart will need to be made to go to the hospital with her.
    - The baby should be monitored by a Doppler during transport.
    - If a tocolytic is available, it should be given to stop the contractions.
    - An IV with normal saline or lactated ringers will need to be started.

6. **Should the cord be replaced into the vagina?** It is best not to handle the cord as this can cause a spasm, completely stopping flow. In cases where a cesarean section cannot be done immediately, the cord can be replaced and the presenting part be pushed down into the pelvis and held there to prevent the cord from prolapsing again. This is not always successful, and valuable time can be lost in doing the procedure. There has been some success with introducing a Foley catheter into the mother's bladder and instilling up to 500 mL of fluid to hold the baby off the cord. A cord outside of the birth canal should be covered with a sterile, warm saline dressing during the transport.

7. **Josie is to be transported to the hospital. How should this transport be accomplished?** Josie must be transported in an ambulance as fast as possible. Time is critical. The midwife cannot remove her hand from holding the presenting part off the baby's cord.

8. **At the hospital Josie is given an emergency cesarean section. (It is less than 30 minutes since she first entered the birth center.) The baby's APGARS are 2 at one minute, 5 at five minutes, and then 6 at ten minutes. The baby is put on a ventilator and admitted to the neonatal intensive care unit. Within eight hours the baby is able to be removed from the ventilator and is doing well. What problems can be anticipated for this baby?** Since this baby was term, the prolapse was identified, and action taken immediately, the baby's chances for recovery are good. Long-term developmental problems cannot be determined until the baby is older. Any baby that required ventilator care is at a higher risk for infection. Stress also increases hypoglycemia and decreases a baby's ability to maintain his temperature. This baby may initially experience some feeding problems.

9. **What problems might the mother experience postpartum?** The mother is at a higher risk for infection and postpartum depression.

References

Simpson, K. R., & Creehan, P. A. (2001). *AWHONN perinatal nursing* (2nd ed.). Philadelphia: Lippincott, Williams & Wilkins.

Varney, H., Kriebs, J., & Gegor, C. (2004). *Varney's midwifery* (4th ed.). Boston: Jones and Bartlett.

Case Study 10: *Jennifer*

1. **What is the role of the doula?** A doula is a labor-support person. Her role is to provide support and comfort measures for the woman and information for her and her family. The positive effects of a doula on labor are evidence-based. Doula-supported labors are faster and have a significantly lower rate of cesarean sections and epidural and forceps deliveries. Maternal satisfaction is also higher when a woman has a doula for support (Hodnett, 2003).

2. **How will the nurse determine if Jennifer's membranes have ruptured?** The nurse can check the fluid with nitrazine paper. If the paper turns a dark blue-green it is probably amniotic fluid. This paper checks the pH. Amniotic fluid is slightly alkaline with a pH~7.15. Vaginal secretions with amniotic fluid will result in a pH from 6.5 to 7.5. False positive values may occur if the mother has vaginal infections that alter the pH or if the specimen is contaminated with blood or with cervical mucus. The nurse may also take a sample of the fluid and check it under a microscope for a ferning pattern. This pattern is also an indication of amniotic fluid.

3. **What is the significance of the findings from the pelvic exam?** Since she is a primigravida, it could be a concern that this baby has not dropped. However she is 36-2/7 weeks gestation and this may account for the fact that lightening has not yet occurred. Primigravidas often will experience lightening (baby dropping deeper in the pelvis) at around 38 weeks gestation.

4. **What is the significance of the ruptured membranes in Jennifer's case?** Spontaneous rupture of membranes and preterm labor may be early indicators of infection. Inflammation processes, such as occur with infections (even those that are asymptomatic), cause disruption of the deciduas and membranes. They can also release prostaglandins. Some vaginal flora produce enzymes that increase the concentration of arachidonic acid (precursor of prostaglandins). Some microorganisms and white blood cells (WBC) also produce a variety of proteolytic enzymes, which break down proteins and may lead to breakdown of mucus plug, rupture of membranes, and entry of bacteria into uterus. Also, ruptured membranes and a high station put the baby at higher risk for prolapsed cord.

5. **What stage of labor is she in?** At admission she is in first stage—the end of the latent phase. Her labor should start to get more active from this point on.

    After six hours Jennifer is 5 cm, 100% effaced, and −3 station. The nurse notes that the baby is in an occiput posterior (OP) presentation. This presentation puts the hard back of the baby's head against the mother's spine. Descent is slower and more painful.

6. **How does the baby's presentation impact the labor?** Labor may be slow and back pain more intense. The smaller posterior fontanel is in the rear segment of the maternal pelvis, and the larger brow and bregma are in the anterior segment. In most cases the baby will rotate anteriorly, and labor will progress. This position is more frequent in the forepelvis that is narrow, such as in the android and anthropoid pelvis. The anthropoid pelvis is common in black women. Progress may arrest, and a cesarean section may become necessary.

7. **What comfort measures might the doula use to help Jennifer cope with the labor?** Any position that takes the pressure of the baby's head off Jennifer's back

will relieve some of the pain. Knee-chest in early labor may help rotate the baby. During the labor the mother may be taught how to do lunges to the side. These are done from a standing position. Kneeling and leaning over a birth ball can be helpful. Counterpressure to the lower back, cold compresses on the lower back, pelvic tilting, and pelvic rock are all helpful. A passive pelvic tilt can be done by the doula while the mother lies on her side. Abdominal lifting may help. To do this the woman, in a standing position, lifts her abdomen with her hands during the contraction. (She lifts the uterus from just above the pubic bone.) At the same time she tilts her pelvis under. She holds the baby up for the entire contraction and then allows him to settle down during the rest period between contractions. This helps to align a baby that may not be well aligned. Stroking the baby in the direction that she wants the baby to turn (to move from an occiput posterior to an occiput anterior presentation) during the contraction may also help (Nichols, 2000). During the pushing stage, she can lie on the side that the occiput is pointing to encourage rotation. One way to increase the natural endorphins to reduce back pain in OP deliveries is to use sterile water papules injected over the sacral area. These "sting," thus increasing the production of local endorphins to the area and will offer approximately one and a half hours of relief. Another way to increase endorphins for back labor relief is to use a transcutaneous electrical nerve stimulator (TENS) unit. This works basically the same as the water papules by increasing local endorphin production and blocking nerve pathways that cause pain. Women who have cardiac pacemakers and those with seizure disorders or undiagnosed sources of pain should not use TENS. Finally, squatting will give more space for the baby to pass through and may be helpful for an OP delivery.

8. **What positions might the mother use to help the baby rotate and descend?** The side-lying position uses the weight of the baby's head to encourage the rotation; hands-and-knees can also be effective in rotating the baby.

   Four hours later the mother is 8 cm, 100% effaced, and −2 station. The baby has rotated to the left occiput transverse (LOT) presentation. This turns the baby to face the mother's side and reduces the pressure on her back.

9. **Jennifer complains that she needs to push. What are the consequences if she were to push at this point?** The cervix may swell, slowing labor. Pushing prior to complete dilatation may also cause tears to the cervix.

   Jennifer does not progress in the next two hours, the baby is developing a large caput, and the FHT are now 150s with an occasional variable deceleration. Contractions are every two minutes, 90 seconds in length, and strong with good relaxation between. The obstetrician expresses concern that he may need to do a cesarean section. Jennifer asks for more time to see if she can begin to progress again.

10. **Which of the following would be appropriate management of Jennifer at this point?**
    a. **The doctor allows her two more hours to dilatate and orders Pitocin to make the contraction more effective.** This is not appropriate since her contractions are already at 90 seconds q 2 minutes and strong; increased stimulation will only cause hyperstimulation and possible fetal distress. Overstressing the uterus can also lead to placenta abruption, uterine rupture, and/or postpartum hemorrhage.

b. **She is given an epidural to help the baby rotate and descend.** An epidural at this time may restrict her movement. This will interfere with the baby's rotation and descent. It may also relax the pelvis, which also interferes with descent. On the other hand, if she is extremely tired and stressed from the contractions, it may allow relaxation and allow her to dilatate.

c. **She is given meperidine (Demerol) 50 mg for pain to help her relax.** She is too close to delivery, and the Demerol would not be appropriate at this time since it may cause respiratory depression of the baby after birth.

d. **Jennifer is given IV antibiotics.** Preterm labor, ruptured membranes, and a rising FHT baseline are all indicators for antibiotics in labor.

e. **The doula helps Jennifer assume a hands-and-knees position.** This would be appropriate since Jennifer is having variable decelerations, which may be associated with cord compression. The hands-and-knees position can be very helpful in relieving this pressure and increasing oxygen delivery to the baby.

References

Blackburn, S. (2003). *Maternal, fetal, and neonatal physiology* (2nd ed.). St. Louis, MO: W. B. Saunders Co.

Eappen, S., & Robbins, D. (2002). Nonpharmacological means of pain relief for labor and delivery. *International Anesthesiology Clinician, 40*(4), 103–114.

Gentz, B. A. (2001). Alternative therapies for the management of pain in labor and delivery. *Clinical Obstetrical Gynecology, 44*(4), 704–732.

Hodnett, E. D., Gates, S., Hofmeyr, G. J., & Sakala, C. (2003). Continuous support for women during childbirth. *The Cochrane Library,* 3. Oxford: Updates Software.

Littleton, L., & Engebretson, J. C. (2002). *Maternal, neonatal, and women's health nursing.* Clifton Park, NY: Thomson Delmar Learning.

Nichols, F., & Humenick, S. (2000). *Childbirth education practice, research, and theory.* Philadelphia: W. B. Saunders Co.

Simkin, P. (2001). *The birth partner* (2nd ed.). Boston: The Harvard Common Press.

Case Study 11:   *Multiple Clients*

1. **There are two RNs and one labor technician on duty tonight. While change of shift report was being given, the following request from the women was received at the nurses' station. At 11:30 p.m.:**

   ■ **Frances is asking for an epidural.**

   ■ **Jeanette wants to take off the electronic fetal monitor and walk around.**

   ■ **Ida wants to get up and use the bathroom.**

   There is also a call from admitting that a new client has just arrived and needs to be brought to the labor unit. The labor unit is expected to send someone to transport her. The clerk at the admission desk said that she seems to be in very active labor. This is her fourth baby.

   Which clients need the most immediate attention? While it is appropriate for a technician to transport a client from admission to the labor unit, this client may be very close to delivery and it would be safer for the RN to transport her. Jeanette is in early labor, her baby is engaged, and her membranes are intact. The technician could be instructed to remove the monitor and assist her to the bathroom. Frances had just been checked and could wait a few minutes while the desk clerk puts in a call for the nurse anesthetist. Prior to Ida going to the bathroom, she should be checked. Although she is a primigravida, it has been two hours since her last VE and she was 6 cm at that time. Her request to use the bathroom may mean that she feels the need for a bowel movement, which could mean she is ready to push.

2. **At 11:50 p.m., while walking around in her room, Jeanette's membranes rupture. The fluid is dark greenish with particles in it. It also has a foul odor. When the nurse checks the baby's heart rate she hears an increase in the fetal heart tones prior to a contraction, a sharp drop, and then a rapid return with the heart tones going above the baseline for a few seconds after the contraction. Describe the nursing actions that are appropriate at this time and give the rationales for each.** The pattern of fetal heart tone deceleration is that of a variable deceleration. This is caused by cord compression. Jeanette should be put to bed and positioned on her side. She should be given oxygen at 10 to 12 liters a minute via a face mask. The description of the fluid indicates that thick meconium is present. The presence of meconium is not unexpected since she is past 40 weeks gestation; however, thick meconium raises risk for meconium aspiration syndrome for the infant. Another concern is the foul odor. The nurse needs to check the mother's temperature frequently as this is a sign of infection (chorionamniotis). The FHT baseline will probably increase in response to an increase in maternal metabolism, which occurs with infection. The physician needs to be notified. The neonatal staff needs to be alerted that they will need to be present at the birth. If she does not have an IV, she will need to have one started in anticipation of antibiotics.

3. **Ida complains that she needs to have a bowel movement. She is irritable and refuses to continue her breathing with her doula. Her legs are shaking and she feels nauseated and begins to vomit. The nurse knows that these are all signs of what?** Transition.

4. **The new client is Julie, MWF, a multigravida admitted to the labor unit at 12 midnight. She is found to be 100% effaced, 9 cm dilatated; and the baby is at +3 station. She tells the nurse that she feels the urge to push. She is also demanding pain medication. How should the nurse respond to this client?** If Julie was given narcotic medications this late in the labor, the baby would experience respiratory depression. The best response would be to notify the physician that delivery is imminent and assist Julie with breathing through the delivery.

5. **At 12:05 a.m. Ida is checked by one of the RNs and found to be 10 cm dilatated, 100% effaced; and the baby is at +1 station. (The fetal heart tones are 130s with accelerations and no decelerations.) She says she is tired and does not feel like pushing. What nursing actions are needed at this time?** Since she does not feel like pushing and the baby's heart tones are excellent, she can be encouraged to rest until she feels like pushing. Evidence-based literature demonstrates that the period of active pushing is the hardest on the baby and can be shortened if the mother is allowed to rest after she is completely dilatated and she feels the urge to push.

6. **Describe the best use of the staffing at 12:10 a.m.** There should be one RN with Jeanette until the fetal heart tones return to normal, and one RN with the physician assisting with Julie's delivery. The technician can monitor Ida until

she feels like pushing. Since Frances is having her labor augmented with Pitocin and is experiencing increasing pain, the RN managing Jeanette needs to also be watching Frances's contractions and the baby's response. If her labor is well-established, the nurse may need to reduce or discontinue the Pitocin for more effective labor (Spiegel, 2004). The technician may help her with her breathing and positioning while waiting for the epidural. A call should be put in to the nursing supervisor for additional staffing. The desk clerk can be calling the neonatal team and the physician and transfer the calls to one of the RNs in the client's room when they go through.

7. **At 12:20 a.m. the technician notifies the RN that Jeanette's fetal heart tones have decreased to 90 bmp for the past one minute and have not returned to the baseline. The nurse has instructed the technician to turn her to her side and start her on oxygen. A call was placed to her doctor 20 minutes ago when her membranes ruptured and meconium was noted. The physician has not returned the call as yet. The fetal heart tones do not improve when she is placed on her side. What nursing actions are required at this time?** Do a VE to check for prolapsed cord and dilatation. If she has not started the IV (usually ordered in standard labor orders), this can be done. Lactated ringers or normal saline should be started and run at a rapid rate. Oxygen should be administered; however, it may take up to 10 minutes before the oxygen level at the placenta is increased. If the physician has not responded and the FHT have not returned to baseline after these interventions, a call to any OB in the hospital should be placed by the nursing supervisor.

8. **The nurse anesthetist arrives to do the epidural for Frances at 12:30 a.m. The anesthetist tells the nurse that she has to get back to surgery as soon as possible and wants to quickly get the epidural started. Prior to the epidural being given, what nursing care needs to be completed?** The maternal blood pressure will need to be monitored frequently due to the possible hypotension related to epidural. If the nurse has not had an opportunity to preload the mother with a bolus of at least 500 mL IV fluid the risk for hypotension is even greater. Because of the very heavy demands on the nursing staff at this time, the nurse may refuse to allow the epidural to be started if:

■ the anesthetist cannot stay with the mother for a reasonable period after starting the epidural to monitor her response

■ additional staff cannot be obtained to monitor the mother

9. **At 12:25 a.m. Jeanette's physician calls. He is on his way to the hospital but is caught in a traffic jam and will be there within 15 minutes. He tells the nurse to have Jeanette prepared for a cesarean section and then to notify the surgical area to prepare for her. What nursing actions need to be done to prepare her for surgery?** She will need an explanation of what is happening and why. If she has not already signed consents for cesarean section, this must also be done. Jeanette will need a Foley catheter. If she does not have an IV, she will need one. She will need to be sent to the operating room area where the surgery is to be performed. She will need an epidural and preload bolus of at least 500 cc of IV fluids. An abdominal prep will be done when she arrives in this area. The neonatal team needs to be called.

10. **Prior to the epidural being started Frances complains about the need to push. The nurse checks her and finds her to be only 8 cm dilatated. What would the**

consequences be if she started to push at this time? If she started pushing at this time, she could cause her cervix to swell, delaying dilatation. There is also the possibility of cervical tears when pushing prior to complete dilatation.

References

Hofmeyr, G. J. (2004). Prophylactic intravenous preloading for regional analgesia in labour. *Cochrane Review.*
http://www.medscape.com/viewarticle/485124?src=search.

Daniel-Spiegel, E., Weiner, Z., et al. (2004). For how long should oxytocin be continued during induction of labour? *BJOG: An International Journal of Obstetrics & Gynaecology, 111*(4), 331–334.

Case Study 12: *Margaret*

1. **Identify three possible causes for her sudden change in condition.** Three possible causes are:
   - Placenta abruption
   - Uterine rupture
   - Amniotic fluid embolism

2. **Could this problem have been identified prior to the actual crisis?** No, amniotic fluid embolisms leading to death are rare. There is some speculation that the condition may occur more frequently; however, the devastating sequence of events that leads to maternal death simply do not occur.

3. **Did Margaret's use of the Jacuzzi tub increase her risk for this complication?** No. There is no evidence that water either with or without the Jacuzzi jets increases any risk in labor.

4. **What labor factors have been associated with amniotic fluid embolism?** Although the exact cause is unknown, some factors have been associated with amniotic fluid embolisms. These are rapid labors, especially those labors with hypertonic contractions usually associated with inductions and augmentations. Artificial and spontaneous rupture of membranes may also trigger this complication. However, in this case Margaret's rapid labor was occurring naturally, not a result of induction.

5. **List, in order, the immediate nursing actions to be taken when Margaret cried out and within the first three minutes that followed.** The nurse's first concerns are basic CPR: maintain an airway (prepare for endotracheal intubation) and ventilation with 100% oxygen for the mother, take steps to control the bleeding to maintain circulatory status, monitor blood pressure (hypotension is secondary to shock), maintain cardiac output, and monitor the baby. To do this the nurse needs to immediately recognize the emergency nature of the events, call stat for physician support, and call to have an operating room prepared. The nurse needs to start several IVs with large bore catheters for blood transfusion (fresh whole blood, packed red blood cells, and/or fresh frozen plasma) as soon as possible before the veins collapse. The nurse should prepare to assist with the insertion of a central line, which will be placed as soon as possible by the physician. Positioning the mother will depend on the degree of respiratory distress she is in. With a pulmonary embolism, an upright position might favor respiratory effort; however, she is bleeding profusely and going into shock

so a supine or even Trendelenberg position may be best. The nurse should anticipate and prepare to administer drugs to stabilize the mother. The physician may call for dopamine (infusion 2–20 mg/kg/minute) to treat the hypotensive shock. Maintaining accurate I&O is important.

6. **On autopsy the precipitating problem identified was an amniotic fluid embolism. The immediate response was sudden hypotension, followed by a placenta abruption leading to hemorrhage, shock, and then disseminated intravascular coagulopathy (DIC). Discuss this sequence of events.** The usual clinical presentation of amniotic fluid embolism is respiratory distress followed by cyanosis and cardiovascular collapse, then hemorrhage, and finally coma. Pulmonary vascular resistance is increased and cardiac output is decreased. Systemic vascular resistance decreases, resulting in rapid development of hypotension.

7. **How frequently do amniotic fluid embolisms occur?** This is a very rare occurrence. It is diagnosed in one out of 30,000 deliveries, and the mortality rate is 50%. However, since it is usually diagnosed at autopsy, some cases may be missed if they do not develop severe complications. It has been suggested that the occurrence of amniotic fluid entering the maternal circulation may not even be rare, but in most cases it does not develop the severe complications seen when it is recognized.

8. **What lab tests should the nurse anticipate that the physician will order immediately?** Critical laboratory testing will include arterial blood gases, CBC, platelet count, fibrinogen, fibrin split products, Pt and PTT, and D-dimer.

9. **List the steps in the neonatal resuscitation.** Dry and position the infant on a firm, warm surface. If not breathing on her own, position properly to establish an open airway, suction the mouth and then the nose, insert endotracheal tube if needed, and if no respirations or heart rate is under 100 beats per minute, establish immediate positive pressure ventilation (PPV) with 100% oxygen. Check heart rate and observe color. If heart rate is less than 60 or between 60 and 80 beats per minute and not rising, begin chest compressions at one ventilation for every three compressions. A full cycle-one ventilation and three chest compressions should be completed in two seconds. Chest compressions should be between ½- to ¾-inch deep on the lower third of the sternum (just below a line drawn between the nipples). Reevaluate the infant after 30 seconds. If the heart rate is above 80, the compressions may be stopped. Ventilations should continue with 100% oxygen until spontaneous respirations are evident. Be prepared to restart ventilations and chest compressions should the infant's heart rate begin to fall.

10. **Margaret was being transferred from a small community hospital to a level-three care center. What is the difference between the levels of maternity care?** Level-one care is for low-risk women and provides basic care. A birth center may be considered a level-one facility. Some hospitals with level-one facilities may do cesarean sections. Level two is an intermediate care facility. Cesarean sections can be done at all level-two facilities, and initial care and even short stay care is available for some high-risk infants. Level-three care is offered at large regional centers, and they offer the most sophisticated intensive care for both high-risk mothers and infants.

References

Bowden, K., Kessler, D., Pinette, M., & Wilson, D. (2003, October). Underwater birth: Missing the evidence or missing the point? *Pediatrics, 112,* 972–973.

Bowen, M., et al. (2002). *Nurses drug guide* (4th ed.). Springhouse, PA: Springhouse Publications.

Cunningham, F. G., Gant, N., Leveno, K., Gilstrap, L., Hauth, J. C., & Wenstrom, K. (2001). *Williams Obstetrics* (21st ed.). Norwalk, CT: Appleton & Lange.

Geissbuhler, V., Eberhard, J. (2000). Waterbirths: a comparative study. *Fetal Diagnosis and Therapy, 15*(5), 291–300.

Part 3: Newborn Case Studies

Case Study 1:   *Baby Nova*

1. **What is the rationale for taking the baby to the nursery for observation after the birth?** Prior to evidence-based studies that examined the importance of keeping the mother and baby together, it was thought that the mother would rest better and the baby be observed more closely if the baby were taken to a nursery for a few hours after birth. The main rationale for this was that the baby's temperature could be unstable after birth and nurses in the nursery were better able to monitor this. Currently, however, evidence-based studies clearly demonstrate that separation of the mother and baby is not advisable. The need to keep mothers and babies together is so important that Lamaze International has listed it as one of the six care practices for normal birth that all centers where birth occurs need to implement. In their position paper they point out that there are evidenced studies that demonstrate that, ". . . interrupting, delaying, or limiting the time that a mother and her baby spend together may have a harmful effect on their relationship and on breastfeeding success. Babies stay warm and cry less, and breastfeeding gets off to a good start, when mothers and their babies have frequent time together beginning at birth. Mothers learn to recognize their babies' needs, responding tenderly and lovingly. A connection that endures a lifetime begins to form" (Crenshaw 2003). Furthermore, infants kept with the mothers maintain their temperatures adequately.

   As a nurse, how can you implement policy changes that reflect current evidence-based practice? Every nurse has the responsibility to keep herself up to date on the growing body of evidence that either supports or disputes current nursing policies. Staff nurses can ask to be included in policy reviews and on committees that write new policies. One good way to stay up to date is to subscribe to the professional nursing journals and review the study results as they become available. Journal clubs within nursing units are another way that staff can stay current. Nursing service educators can bring new studies to the attention of the staff and administration. It is important that every nurse view the need for keeping her practice current as a personal responsibility and not accept nor continue policies that do not reflect the current standards. Many policies are based on "common sense" or individual case reviews, and when they are challenged by evidence-based studies they cannot be justified. Separating the mother and baby after a normal birth is just one example of a policy that does not reflect good nursing care.

2. **Why is Baby Nova given first sterile water and then 5% glucose feedings in the nursery?** There is no evidence-based reason for this practice. In addition,

giving a breastfed baby a bottle of anything delays breastfeeding and may increase chances of nipple confusion and make breastfeeding difficult.

3. **Why do you think the baby will not feed when her mother offers her the breast?** This baby just ate a short time ago and may be sleepy from the Stadol, and because she has had a bottle as her first feeding, the manner in which she takes the nipple into her mouth and controls the flow of milk has been imprinted for a bottle. This makes subsequent breastfeedings difficult.

4. **What is happening when the baby looks away from the breast while the mother tries to direct her to the breast?** The baby is rooting toward the mother's hand trying to find the breast. Direct the mother to touch the baby's cheek with the nipple to encourage the baby to turn toward the nipple.

5. **How does the pain medication given the mother affect her attempt to breastfeed at this time?** The baby may be sleepy for several hours after the mother has received Stadol in labor.

6. **Describe proper positioning at the breast for breastfeeding.** The baby should lie directly facing the mother, "tummy to tummy." There is also the cradle hold and the football hold. In all cases, the baby's body and head should be in alignment without turning the head. The baby should rest her head on the mother's forearm, not at the elbow. This puts the baby at the breast at a position that allows the baby to nurse without the breast blocking the baby's nose and without pulling unevenly at the nipple.

7. **Name three things that should have been done differently that would have increased this mother's ability to breastfeed this baby.** The nurse should have assisted the mother to immediately breastfeed after the birth. The mother and baby should not have been separated. The baby should not have been given a bottle of any type, nor given formula. If the mother could have avoided pain medication, the baby would have nursed better. If the mother had received consistent, individualized support in labor, such as use of a doula, she might not have needed the pain medication.

8. **How can the nurse assist her now?** The nurse needs to encourage the mother to build her confidence in her ability to produce adequate milk. Offering formula only undermines this. She needs to be taught the signs of hunger so that she can respond to her baby adequately. Explain supply and demand and the baby's normal reflexes that assist her to feed, such as rooting, sucking, and swallowing. Teach her how to help the baby latch on and how to remove the baby from the breast without traumatizing the nipple.

9. **What are the consequences of giving the baby formula?** Once a breastfeeding mother begins to supplement with formula, the likelihood of continued breastfeeding is greatly decreased. The baby will nurse less because her hunger has been satisfied. Less nursing means less milk production. Nipple confusion can also occur once the infant has been given a bottle. Formula given to an infant prior to six months has been associated with multiple health risks, including increased infections and obesity.

10. **The mother asks, "How long should I breastfeed?" What is the most appropriate answer?** The American Academy of Pediatrics recommends breastfeeding for at least one year.

References

American Academy of Pediatrics. (2005, February). Policy statement: Breastfeeding and the use of human milk. *Pediatrics, 115*(2), 496–506.

Anderson, G. C., Moore, E., Hepworth, J., & Bergman, N. (2003). Early skin-to-skin contact for mothers and their healthy newborn infants. *The Cochrane Library,* 3. Oxford: Update Software.

Biancuzzo, M. (2003). *Breastfeeding the newborn: Clinical strategies for nurses* (2nd ed.). St. Louis, MO: Mosby.

Crenshaw, J., et al. (2003). Case practices that support normal birth: No separation of the mother and baby after birth. *Lamaze International Education Council.* http://normalbirth.lamaze.org/institute/CarePractices/NoSeparation.asp.

Riordan, J., & Auerbach, K. (2005). *Breast feeding and human lactation* (3rd ed.). Sudbury, MA: Jones and Bartlett.

Uvnas-Moberg, K. (1998). Oxytocin may mediate the benefits of positive social interactions and emotions. *Psychoneuro-endocrinology, 23*(8), 819–838.

Case Study 2:   *Baby Haley*

1. **What is Baby's Haley's initial APGAR score?** The baby's APGAR is 5. **List the points for each component.**

	Respiratory Effort	Heart Rate	Tone	Reflex Irritability	Color
2 points	Crying	> or = 100	Active	Cry or cough	Completely pink
1 point	Slow, irregular	<100	Some flexion	Grimace	Pink body, blue extremities
No points	Absent	Absent	Limp	No response	Pale or bluish

2. **The mother was not screened for congenital anomalies. What might the reason be for this?** She started her prenatal care late. She was not considered a high risk. If she had desired screening or was thought to be high risk, she could have had an amniocentesis. It takes 10 to 14 days for the karyotyping to be completed after the amniocentesis is done. High-risk factors would have been age over 35, family history of anomalies, known consanguinity in the parents, or a previous child with anomalies. None of these factors were present in this pregnancy.

3. **What congenital defects would the nurse suspect from the observed characteristics?** The most serious are cardiac anomalies, duodenal atresia, esophageal atresia, and imperforate anus.

4. **How diagnostic are these observations?** This baby has many of the characteristics of trisomy 21 or Down syndrome. However compelling as these observations are, they aren't sufficient to be diagnostic. The baby will need a chromosomal screen before a diagnosis can be confirmed.

5. **If the mother had started prenatal care earlier and had had a triple screen at 18 weeks gestation, what is the possibility that Down syndrome would have been identified?** A triple screen (AFP, unconjugated estriol, and hCG) will identify 60% of Down syndrome babies. Adding inhibin A (quad screen) increases

detection of Down syndrome by approximately 7%. False positive results from these screens are high and are usually due to incorrect gestational age calculation or other factors that influence results, such as diabetes, obesity, multiple gestations, and race.

6. **If the triple screen or quad screen had come back positive for Down syndrome, what further testing would have been recommended?** Further testing includes amniocentesis and high-resolution ultrasound. Complications from amniocentesis occur in approximately .5% or 1 out of 200 procedures. They can be serious, resulting in pregnancy loss. Ultrasound screening may be done for fetal nuchal translucency, and additional ultrasound markers (although still controversial) include choroid plexus cyst, echogenic bowel, echogenic intracardiac focus, and dilitation of the kidneys (pyelctasis). It is important to note that these findings are sometimes found in normal fetuses.

7. **List the special observations that the nurse will make on Baby Haley during his transition.** This baby will need to be observed for signs of cardiac anomalies. Babies with Down syndrome have a 40% chance of having cardiac defects. The most common defect in these babies is a ventricular septal defect. A murmur is not usually detected at birth but will become apparent at around three days of age. These babies may develop congestive heart failure, and about half of them will require surgery. The baby will need to be carefully observed when feedings are attempted. It will be very important to note the passage of meconium.

8. **The mother wants to nurse her son right after delivery. How should the nurse respond?** The nurse should encourage and help her. Breastfeeding is especially beneficial for this baby. The unique protection from infection afforded by breastfeeding can make a critical difference to these babies. Bonding is very important. Baby Haley may have problems latching on and coordinating sucking and swallowing. His large tongue may make nursing difficult. The baby's tongue may fall to the back of his mouth. Hypotonia may make it difficult for the baby to achieve an adequate seal and to position the baby. The baby can be propped firmly with a pillow in the mother's lap or supported in a sling to free up the mother's hand to steady the jaw and breast. The nurse should contact the lactation consultant immediately and have her meet with the mother during recovery if possible. If Baby Haley cannot coordinate sucking and swallowing, the mother can be assisted and encouraged to pump her breast milk to be given to the baby through a feeding tube.

9. **Baby Haley's mother asks the nurse, "What is wrong with him? My daughter seemed so different at birth." How should the nurse respond?** The nurse needs to be sensitive to the mother's observations and acknowledge them. Using terms such as "special baby" may be helpful. At this time a diagnosis should not be assigned to the baby. The nurse can discuss the need for further diagnostic testing and focus on the immediate needs of the baby. Most important is that the nurse listen to the mother and encourage contact between the mother, father, and baby.

10. **The father walks out of the delivery room, sits in a chair in the hall, and puts his head in his hands and cries. How should the nurse approach him?** As with the mother, the baby's father will need someone to listen to him, confirm his observations, and discuss plans for the immediate testing and care of the baby.

He should be encouraged, but not forced, to hold his son and spend time with his wife and baby. The nurse can point out the normal characteristics, e.g., if the baby responds to a loud sound, the nurse can point out this response.

References

Baliff, J. P., & Mooney, R. A. (2003, December). New developments in prenatal screening for Down syndrome. *American Journal of Clinical Pathology, 120,* S14–24.

Biancuzzo, M. (2003). *Breastfeeding the newborn: Clinical strategies for nurses* (2nd ed.). St. Louis, MO: Mosby.

Brigatti, K. W., & Malone, F. D. (2004, March). First-trimester screening for aneuploidy. *Obstetrical Gynecology Clinic of North America, 31*(1), 1–20.

Blackburn, S. (2003) *Maternal, fetal, and neonatal physiology* (2nd ed.). St. Louis, MO: W. B. Saunders Co.

Lawrence, R., & Lawrence, R. (1999). *Breastfeeding: a guide for the medical profession.* St. Louis, MO: Mosby.

Morris, K. (2004, April). *Prenatal screening for birth defects: an update. Missouri Medicine, 101*(2), 121–124.

Riordan, J., & Auerbach, K. (2005). *Breast feeding and human lactation* (3rd ed.). Sudbury, MA: Jones and Bartlett.

Tappero, E., & Honeyfield, M. E. (2003). *Physical assessment of the newborn* (3rd ed.). Petaluma, CA: NICU Ink.

Case Study 3:   *Baby Maria*

1. **How might the fact that Baby Maria was born by a cesarean section impact on her mother's ability to be successful at breastfeeding?** Baby Maria's mother will experience increased postpartum pain and there will be increased separation of mother and baby. Pain and pain medications, difficulty moving about, IVs with possible antibiotics, and an increased need to monitor the mother and baby will interfere with the normal transition of the mother to her new role. Nursing efforts need to be directed toward reducing these obstacles. The baby should be brought to her mother frequently. An even better arrangement would be to arrange for 24-hour rooming in with a family member encouraged to stay with the mother to help her care for Baby Maria in the room (American Academy of Pediatrics & American College of Obstetricians and Gynecologists, 2002). The mother should have special assistance with breastfeeding. The nurse should be certain that there is an early visit from the lactation consultant to provide anticipatory guidance and support for the breastfeeding. A postpartum doula may be helpful.

2. **What are the implications of Baby Maria being supplemented with formula at night?** This is often done when the mother has had a cesarean section. Although breastfed babies who receive any other form of feeding have twice the infection rate as babies who are totally breastfed, the breastfeeding will still provide some protection from infection from the increased antibodies passed from the mother to the baby. Missing breastfeedings decreases stimulation to the mother's breast, which will slow the process of milk production. This makes it more difficult for the mother to build her initial milk supply. Increased feedings can overcome this if night supplement feedings are not continued or increased. When the hospital supplements breastfed babies with formula

feedings, there is a much higher incidence of mothers who do not continue to breastfeed. The mother's level of confidence in her ability to breastfeed is undermined.

3. **How should the nurse respond to the mother's request for formula?** It is common today for a young mother to have never held a newborn prior to her own and to never even have watched a newborn being breastfed. This lack of experience and overwhelming bombardment by the formula culture has left her unprepared to breastfeed. Consistent commercial exposure by formula advertising deludes young women into thinking that formula is an ideal food for their babies. While there are rare cases where a woman cannot breastfeed, 97% of women are capable of doing so without any supply problems. Educating the mother on supply and demand is critical to building her confidence in her ability to feed her baby. The nurse should not bring a bottle to the mother. The nurse should take the time to sit with the mother, discuss milk production, and discourage any supplemental feedings. Consistent, frequent exclusive breastfeeding will increase the mother's milk production. By pointing out how formula is deficient in the immuno-complements that protect her baby and how breast milk is better digested by the baby, the nurse can discourage giving the baby further formula. Another reason to discourage continued supplementation is that the baby may become used to taking milk from a bottle and will begin to reject the mother's nipple since she will have to suck differently and harder. This is called nipple confusion. Convincing the mother not to continue supplementation will be difficult since the staff has already introduced this baby to the bottle at night. Furthermore, formula samples and coupons given to the mother to take home have been strongly associated with early weaning. To help Maria and other mothers have more successful breastfeeding experiences, the nurse may work to establish firm policies that discourage supplementation and take-home formula.

4. **What suggestions might the nurse give to increase the mother's milk supply?** The most significant one is to have the mother feed frequently and not continue to supplement feedings at night. Drinking adequate fluids is also important. The mother should be encouraged to drink to thirst. The practice of assigning a set amount of fluid to drink is not advised since overhydration may interfere with letdown. The mother should be aware of her thirst and arrange to have a glass of fluid at each breastfeeding.

5. **What positions might the nurse assist the mother to sit or lie in that will make her more comfortable for nursing after a cesarean section?** Because the mother's abdomen is tender after the major surgery, she can be taught to hold the baby in the football hold with a pillow to support the baby's weight. She may try to nurse lying on her side. Both interventions will keep the weight of the baby off her incision. The baby should lie so that her abdomen is toward the mother. This will position the baby to approach the breast directly head-on. When the baby has to turn her head to come to the breast, she pulls the nipple unevenly, which may cause sore, cracked nipples.

6. **Explain the most probable cause of the "white spots on Maria's nose and chin"?** This is probably milia, a normal variation seen on most babies. Milia results from blocked sebaceous glands and should be left alone. The condition will clear on its own.

7. **How should the nurse explain the "bruises" on the baby's buttocks and legs?** Latin, Native American, and dark-colored babies often have Mongolian spots on their lower backs, buttocks, and upper thighs. These are harmless variations and will fade over time. It is important that the parents understand that these are not bruises because they sometimes look like them. They should be recorded in the baby's chart to avoid mistaken diagnosis of abuse later.

8. **What explanation can the nurse give for the condition of the baby's feet?** The bluish color is called acrocyanosis and is a common finding within the first 24 hours. Peripheral circulation lags behind central circulation while the baby adjusts to life outside the uterus.

9. **Maria's mom is getting meperidine hydrochloride (Demerol) for pain relief. How can the nurse help Baby Maria's mother to relax and achieve the most effect from less medication?** The Demerol may make the baby sleepy. To provide the mother the most relief and avoid the sleepy response in the baby, the medication should be given immediately after the breastfeeding. This allows the mother's system an opportunity to process and eliminate much of the drug and its metabolites prior to the next feeding. Also, if the nurse takes time to make sure that the mother is comfortable by eliminating environmental noise and excessive or irritating light, taking time to help her relax, arranging her pillows to support her well, and making sure that she has something to drink at the bedside when administering pain medication, the mother will benefit from its effects longer and request less overall medication. Today, when there is so much emphasis on pain relief, it is important that the nurse understand that encouraging pain medications is not the only way to reduce pain, especially in the new mother. Furthermore, nurses need to recognize the potential detrimental effects of pain medications on maternal long-term goals.

References

American Academy of Pediatrics. (2005, February). Policy statement: Breastfeeding and the use of human milk. *Pediatrics, 115*(2), 496–506.

American Academy of Pediatrics (AAP) and American College of Obstetricians and Gynecologists (ACOG). (2002). *Guidelines for perinatal care.* Elk Grove Village, IL: ACOG.

Freda, M. (2002). *Perinatal patient education.* Philadelphia: Lippincott, Williams & Wilkins.

Littleton, L., & Engebretson, J. C. (2002). *Maternal, neonatal, and women's health nursing.* Clifton Park, NY: Thomson Delmar Learning.

Case Study 4:   *Baby James*

1. **What is the significance of the fact that this mother had no prenatal care?** One of the major concerns at this point is determining the gestational age of the newborn. The most accurate way of doing this is by examining the infant's physical characteristics. It also would have been helpful if a date had been determined early in the antepartum period. This dating process is important because it helps to predict the current maturity of the fetus at the estimated date of delivery. The infant's lungs are usually mature by 35 weeks; but if her dates are wrong, this baby could be at high risk for several complications related to prematurity such as respiratory distress syndrome, hypothermia, and hypoglycemia. In addition, the maternal information is not known such as

patterns of fetal growth, overall maternal health during the pregnancy, any pregnancy complications that developed, and maternal screening and diagnostic lab work including blood type and GBS status, rubella immune status, hepatitis and HIV status, and information on history and/or current sexually transmitted infections.

2. **What are the risks involved in a precipitous delivery?** A precipitous delivery may cause trauma to both the mother in the form of cervical and vaginal tears and to the infant including cephalohematoma and different types of palsy.

3. **What do you think might have been done differently for this delivery had the mother come in at 4 to 6 cm instead of 9 cm?** Rupture of membranes greater than 16 hours, especially prior to term, is a major risk factor for both mother and baby. The longer the duration of membrane rupture, the greater the risk of developing an infection known as chorioamnionitis. This problem coupled with prematurity, especially considering that there was no prenatal care, is indication for routine prophylactic antibiotics during labor. An additional warning sign of maternal–fetal infection is the baby's tachycardic fetal heart baseline.

4. **List the progressive signs of respiratory distress exhibited by this infant after birth.** The classic signs of respiratory distress in an infant are tachypnea (over 60 breaths/minute), nasal flaring, grunting, and sternal retractions. These are early signs of respiratory distress due to any etiology and are usually exhibited prior to the development of central cyanosis. Remember, central cyanosis with respiratory distress is a very ominous sign and should be considered an emergency. Cyanosis without respiratory distress is suggestive of congenital heart disease and needs further assessment.

5. **This baby is initially being screened for infection and treated for transient tachypnea of the newborn (TTN). What data supports this diagnosis?** This baby had a good five-minute APGAR score but then exhibited a rapid respiratory rate or tachypnea. Transient tachypnea of the newborn or RDS type II is a benign condition of the near term or the larger term infants. It is the result of delayed reabsorption of amniotic fluid from the baby's lungs, a mild degree of lung immaturity, and dilution of surfactant that is present by the residual amniotic fluid. Infants who are delivered via a cesarean section are at increased risk of developing TTN because of the lack of stress such as that experienced in a vaginal birth. The absence of this stress results in lower fetal catecholamine increase than that experienced in a vaginal birth. The catecholamine increase serves to mature the lungs and aids in the lymphatic absorption of the remaining amniotic fluid from the lungs. Additionally, in a cesarean section the normal squeeze of the fetal chest as the baby progresses down the birth canal and recoil that occurs in a vaginal birth do not occur. These mechanical changes also serve to clear the infant's lungs. Immediately after birth, many babies will have some of these symptoms, which are transient in nature and should resolve spontaneously. The continuation of any of these symptoms beyond 20 to 30 minutes of life indicates the development of a more serious condition such as early onset of sepsis and/or respiratory distress syndrome. This infant's physical assessment at six hours of age clearly supports the diagnosis of the serious type I form of respiratory distress syndrome. With the facts that the due date was not well established prior to birth and that the baby was found to be preterm along with progressive development of respiratory distress, some hypoglycemia, and

persistent temperature instability, the nurse should have recognized that this baby needed immediate attention. By failing to call the physician to have the baby transferred, the nurse may have placed the baby in additional jeopardy. This baby should have been transported to the neonatal intensive care unit (NICU) during the transitional period after about 30 minutes when the respiratory distress became progressively worse.

6. **What is the most likely reason for this baby's initial hypoglycemia?** Stress during the labor as evidenced by the tachycardia, the baby's precipitous delivery, and the sudden environmental change all combined to increase the infant's metabolism and glucose utilization significantly. This infant is having trouble maintaining his temperature because of prematurity, the development of respiratory distress, and the possibility that there may be an infection present. The normal infant response to hypothermia is to increase heat production by increasing basal metabolism. A drop of only 1°F will increase glucose needs by two times. It is important to remember that there is often a normal period of relative hypoglycemia that occurs in the first hour of life; this should be transient in nature. Hypoglycemia becomes much more of an issue with respiratory distress or in the preterm or some of the larger full-term infants. Persistent hypoglycemia below the level 40 for more than an hour leads to the potential for brain damage that is inversely proportional to the degree of hypoglycemia.

7. **Assess the baby's vital signs. Which ones are within normal range and which ones need attention?** Respiratory rate is too rapid, temperature is too low, and heart rate is within normal limits.

8. **List the risk factors that existed for infection.** Factors that increase risk for infection for this baby are:
   - Premature and prolonged rupture of membranes
   - Preterm delivery
   - Precipitous delivery
   - No prenatal care
   - Unknown GBS status

9. **Why is this baby hypothermic, and how does it affect this baby's transition?** There are several possible reasons why this baby cannot maintain his temperature. He has experienced one of several sources of cold stress during the early transition period and resuscitation. These stressors include radiation to the relatively cold environment, convection from the circulating air conditioning, conduction from any cold blankets, and evaporation from inadequate drying and cold oxygen flowing across his face. Once the temperature drops, babies must work harder metabolically to raise their temperatures back to within normal limits since infants do not shiver as adults do. This increase in metabolic activity directly affects the infant's glucose utilization, which in turn helps to support the temperature stability. Preterm infants have limited glucose stores because their brown and yellow fat deposits have not been completed, and this further reduces their ability to warm themselves. One of the purposes of the yellow fat is to insulate infants from the cold stress of the extrauterine environment. The brown fat is utilized for energy and to maintain temperature. Baby James must increase his metabolism to bring his temperature up. This metabolic increase requires more oxygen and depletes his glucose stores. This increase in oxygen demand from combined effects of the respiratory distress, the

different types of cold stresses, and the lack of energy stores all together make the baby's oxygen delivery inadequate for the complete metabolic processes of burning fat. This metabolic deficiency leads to the development of a metabolic acidosis. A further complication of hypothermia is that it interferes with surfactant production, making the transition to extrauterine life even more difficult. Surfactant is necessary to maintain lung function and prevent atelectasis. Respiratory distress, hypothermia, and inability to maintain temperature, especially in the preterm baby, are all hallmark signs that this baby may be developing infection. In other words, the hypothermic baby, with or without respiratory distress, is septic until proven otherwise.

10. **How significant is the acrocyanosis?** Acrocyanosis is cyanosis that occurs distally in one or more of the baby's extremities. By itself this is a very common variation, is a sign of transient vasomotor instability, and usually resolves spontaneously. But in combination with the other signs of respiratory difficulty, it may be more significant. The nurse needs to determine if central cyanosis is also present, which would indicate a more serious problem.

11. **What is the significance of jaundice in a six-hour-old infant?** This is also known as hyperbilirubinemia. Prior to 24 hours, jaundice is abnormal even in the premature infant. It is a well-known fact that preterm infants have increased incidence of jaundice, but it should not be this early. Early hyperbilirubinemia is often associated with an infection or some type of blood incompatibility such as Rh or ABO setups. If the level of hyperbilirubinemia rises above a critical level, this preterm baby is at risk for central nervous system depression, poor feeding, and the rare possibility of brain damage from kernicterus if the bilirubin crosses the blood–brain barrier in significant levels.

References

Blackburn, S. (2003). *Maternal, fetal, and neonatal physiology* (2nd ed.). St. Louis, MO: W. B. Saunders Co.

Littleton, L., & Engebretson, J. C. (2002). *Maternal, neonatal, and women's health nursing.* Clifton Park, NY: Thomson Delmar Learning.

Simpson, K. R., & Creehan, P. A. (2001). *AWHONN perinatal nursing* (2nd ed.). Philadelphia: Lippincott, Williams & Wilkins.

Case Study 5:   *Baby Ittybit*

1. **From an initial assessment, what is the main problem in this situation?** The grandmother is the problem. Many grandmothers today bottle-fed their infants and lack any understanding of the breastfeeding process. It is difficult for some of these women to have to learn that they were misled about the benefits of formula feeding and that the quality of breast milk is superior to formula. A generation ago families were told by the commercial formula makers that formula was superior to breast milk, and the majority chose to bottle-feed. Today many of their college-educated daughters have discovered that there are no formulas on the market, even today, that can compare favorably to breast milk. Recently the U.S. Department of Health and Human Services has started a major campaign, the National Breastfeeding Awareness Campaign, to inform

parents about the benefits of breastfeeding and the risks of formula feeding. The Healthy People 2010 health objectives address increasing breastfeeding among minority populations, stating Blacks as one population that needs encouragement. These daughters choose to breastfeed, but their families are not prepared to support them and often unwittingly undermine their confidence with false information.

2. **What is the most probable explanation for the baby being jaundiced?** Newborn physiologic jaundice begins to peak from 48 to 72 hours after birth. It is the result of the infant reducing his hemoglobin level to a level that is normal for extrauterine life. **Give supporting evidence for your answer.** The baby is 48 hours old, eating well, and is alert and active.

3. **Explain the physiology of physiologic jaundice.** Babies have more red blood cells than they need after birth. The process of breaking down excessive RBC releases bilirubin into the circulation. Since the liver is the organ that processes (conjugates) the bilirubin to prepare it to leave the body and it is still immature at birth, bilirubin may concentrate in the blood at high enough levels that it becomes visible as a yellow color of the skin and mucus membranes. This yellow color is known as jaundice and becomes visible when the levels of indirect or direct bilirubin reach around 2 to 4 mg/dL (Morrow Cavanaugh, 1999). The baby does not take in a large quantity of fluid during the early days of breastfeeding. This slight dehydration may make it harder for the baby to clear the bilirubin. However, much of the bilirubin is excreted from the body through the gut (stool). Breastfed babies have the advantage of a laxative effect from the colostrum and early breast milk, which helps to clear the jaundice. Mothers should be encouraged to breastfeed more often and not supplement with water or formula.

4. **Baby Ittybit is Black American. How is jaundice assessed in darker skinned infants?** Dark skinned babies may be assessed for jaundice by checking the sclera of the eyes, by checking their mucus membranes, and by pressing down over the sternum.

5. **Explain how breast milk affects neonatal jaundice.** See the answer to question 3 about dehydration. Breast milk jaundice on the other hand has nothing to do with the technique of feeding and is probably related to an enzyme in the mother's milk that allows for a greater absorption of unconjugated bilirubin, causing a prolonged and high level of jaundice (Biancuzzo, 2003). This usually will not happen until at least 5 to 7 days. When jaundice related to breastfeeding does occur, there is never a serious threat to the baby and he or she will outgrow it shortly. Some pediatricians ask the mother to stop breastfeeding for a few feedings (supplement with formula) to observe if the bilirubin goes down. If it does, that confirms that breast milk was the cause of the jaundice, and the mother can then go right back to breastfeeding without worries about the jaundice. Breast milk jaundice is self-limiting and will clear spontaneously. Stopping breastfeeding is really not necessary and exposes the baby unnecessarily to formula. Formula feeding reduces the protection from infection provided by breast milk. Formula interferes with the process of gut sealing that occurs with exclusive breast milk. Formula also alters the intestinal pH to favor bacteria growth. A baby who is active, alert, and feeding well is not having a problem with pathologic jaundice.

6. **Is it probable that breast milk is the problem?** No, it is too early for this type of jaundice to be a problem. **Why or why not?** Breast milk jaundice occurs after 5 to 7 days or more. This baby is only 48 hours old, is active and alert, and probably has physiologic jaundice.

7. **What observations can the nurse make that will help determine if the baby is experiencing pathologic jaundice?** Is the baby eating well? Is he alert and active when awake? Does the baby wake up on his own every two to three hours to feed? Does the baby have good muscle tone?

8. **List four causes of pathologic jaundice.**
   - Infection
   - Blood incompatibility
   - Bile duct blockage
   - Any liver problem
   - Internal bleeding

9. **Describe the four steps of bilirubin metabolism.**
   1. Production of bilirubin (the breakdown of the RBC) **1.**
   2. Transport (movement of the bilirubin throughout the bloodstream usually bound to albumin, which keeps it out of the CNS)
   3. Clearance in the liver (conjugation—this makes the bilirubin water soluble and prepares it to be excreted)
   4. Recirculation (This occurs in the gut when for some reason the baby does not excrete it. It becomes unconjugated and then starts the process all over again.)

10. **What are the potential consequences if Baby Ittybit has pathologic jaundice and it is not treated?** Pathologic jaundice can lead to central system damage (kernicterus) and even death.

11. **Outline a teaching plan to educate the parents and grandmother about jaundice and to empower the mother on her ability to make decisions about her baby's care.**
    - Teach normal feeding and sleeping patterns of the neonate
    - Teach benefits of breastfeeding
    - Teach stooling patterns of the breastfed neonate
    - Recommend taking the baby in the sun for short periods to help reduce the jaundice (without too much direct sun exposure)
    - Reinforce the mother's knowledge about her baby

References

American Academy of Pediatrics. *Breastfeeding initiatives at the American academy of pediatrics.* http://www.aap.org/healthtopics/breastfeeding.cfm.

American Academy of Pediatrics. (2005, February). Policy statement: Breastfeeding and the use of human milk. *Pediatrics, 115*(2), 496–506.

Biancuzzo, M. (2003). *Breastfeeding the newborn* (2nd ed.). St. Louis, MO: Mosby.

Blackburn, S. (2003). *Maternal, fetal, and neonatal physiology* (2nd ed.). St. Louis, MO: W. B. Saunders Co.

Littleton, L., & Engebretson, J. C. (2002). *Maternal, neonatal, and women's health nursing.* Clifton Park, NY: Thomson Delmar Learning.

Morrow Cavanaugh, B. (1999). *Nurses manual of laboratory and diagnostic tests* (3rd ed.). Philadelphia: F. A. Davis.

National Breastfeeding Awareness Campaign. (2004). http://4woman.gov.

Case Study 6: *Baby Chary*

1. **The mother stated that she never missed a birth control pill. What is the possibility of getting pregnant while not missing any pills?** When a woman follows instructions perfectly, never missing a pill, the chances of her getting pregnant are 1 in 1000. The pregnancy rate does increase to 1 in 20 or 5% if there is a history of her forgetting to take a pill at times. She was also taking minocycline, which may have decreased the effectiveness of her birth control pill and increased her risks of becoming pregnant.

2. **What are the risks to the baby since the mother continued to take the birth control pill for the first two months of her pregnancy?** Most long-term studies of women who took the pill during the early months of pregnancy do not show any adverse effects on the fetus. One study did indicate a possibility of increased incidence of urinary tract problems in these babies (Li De-Kun, 1995).

3. **The mother asks the nurse what the pink mark is on her baby's neck. The nurse examines the mark and finds that it is small, approximately 1 cm flat with irregular edges. It blanches with pressure, and becomes darker as the baby cries. How should the nurse reply to the mother?** This is called a nevus simplex and is sometimes called a stork bite. It will usually last one or two years and then just gradually fade; at times it disappears on its own. It is very common, and there are no other problems associated with it.

4. **The mother notices that the baby does not seem to hear her. When and how will the baby's hearing be checked?** The baby's hearing will be checked before discharge from the hospital. State law often mandates such screening. The baby's hearing will be checked by either the evoked otoacoustic emission test (EOAE) or the auditory brainstem response (ABR). The EOAE measures sound waves in the inner ear. The ABR measures electroencephalographic waves recorded by an electrode placed on the newborn's forehead. Both of these screening techniques are non-invasive, safe, and accurate. If there is a problem identified, the infant will be referred to a specialist for a full hearing test.

5. **Review the medications that the mother took for the acne. What possible consequences do they present for the infant?** The minocycline is a tetracycline and is pregnancy classification D. If used in the second half of the pregnancy, it may cause damage to the infant's permanent teeth and bones. Even primary teeth may be stained. The erythromycin-benzoyl peroxide gel (Benzamycin topical gel) is a category B.

6. **What is the significance of the skin tag on the baby's right ear?** Skin tags are usually benign, but since the baby also has a preauricular sinus these may be indications of internal ear anomalies. The presence of either one of these findings would mandate an otoscopic exam and hearing screen and may require a renal ultrasound since there is a slightly increased possibility of renal abnormalities in the presence of aural anomalies.

7. **On day three the pediatrician decided to look at the baby's ear canal with an otoscope. Describe how this procedure is done.** This is often delayed until the baby is a few days old to allow time for the vernix, mucus, blood, and amniotic fluid to drain from the ear canal. During the exam, the baby must be wrapped securely to keep the baby from moving, and the otoscope is used to view the

tympanic membrane by pulling the pinna back and down. This examination is also done if an infection is suspected, which is rare in the neonatal period.

8. **What are the advantages to early detection of hearing loss?** Early detection of any hearing defect can allow for early intervention to minimize any future speech, language, or cognitive problems that can occur. In many states, it is mandatory for all newborns.

9. **Discuss the mother's illness in the second trimester and her taking the azithromycin (Zithromax) at that time.** In most cases, second trimester exposure to medications is less dangerous than first trimester exposure since the fetal organogenesis is completed. Sinus infections can often be very painful and sometimes dangerous. Azithromycin (Zithromax) is a pregnancy class B drug. The risk to the fetus from the exposure to a category B drug is far less than the benefit gained by the mother in taking it in this case. Baby Chary should not be at an increased risk from this drug exposure. Depending on the organisms that caused the sinus infection, the baby may be at risk from that exposure; but this is almost impossible to determine.

10. **How does Trichomonas vaginitis affect pregnancy? How safe is metronidazole (Flagyl) in the third trimester?** Trichomonas vaginitis is a sexually transmitted illness and has been associated with preterm labor. If present, it is treated during the second and third trimesters. Metronidazole (Flagyl) is given orally and considered to be a category B medication and is usually safe during the latter trimesters. Metronidazole (Flagyl) may also be given vaginally, but it is less effective by that route and may induce premature rupture of membranes. Metronidazole (Flagyl) vaginal preparations should not be used in pregnancy.

11. **Discuss the mother's use of tobacco and nicotine. Is Baby Chary at increased risk for any health problems because of it?** Smoking in pregnancy is associated with decreased fetal growth leading to small-for-gestational-age (SGA) babies, placenta abruption, and changes in FHT. Because the mother was able to quit by her fourth month, many of these risk are minimized. It is important that she be counseled not to start again, as neonatal exposure can also increase health risks to the newborn such as infection and reactive airway disease, sudden infant death syndrome (SIDS), and upper respiratory tract infections.

References

Blackburn, S. (2003). *Maternal, fetal, and neonatal physiology* (2nd ed.). St Louis, MO: W. B. Saunders Co.

Li, De-Kun, Daling, J. R., Mueller, B. A., Hickok, D. E., Fantel, A. G., & Weiss, N.S. (1995). Oral contraceptive use after conception in relation to the risk of congenital urinary tract anomalies. *Teratology, 51,* 30–36.

Simpson, K. R., & Creehan, P. A. (2001). *AWHONN perinatal nursing* (2nd ed.). Philadelphia: Lippincott, Williams & Wilkins.

Case Study 7:   *Baby Cunningham*

1. **What is the most likely cause of this infant's distress?** By physical examination, Baby Cunningham is between 32 to 33 weeks gestation and large for gestational age at greater than the 95th percentile. Because of this prematurity, the lack of

mature surfactant contributes to respiratory distress syndrome type I. This baby also lacked the normal physiologic squeeze that occurs during vaginal delivery, making it difficult for her to clear her lungs and maintain normal respirations.

2. **List the dangers of elective induction.** There are many dangers of elective induction. The most obvious one is that the uterus is not ready for labor and the induction will fail, resulting in a cesarean section. In the past few years, it was found that the use of prostaglandins could ripen a cervix and allow for inductions prior to signs of uterine preparedness. The use of oxytocin with prostaglandins has been associated with an increased incidence of uterine rupture and fetal distress due to hyperstimulation, amniotic embolism, and the possibility of inducing the delivery of a preterm infant, especially if the baby is large for gestational age. One major problem with the latter issue is unexpected prematurity and that a premature baby will be delivered with complications related to the prematurity. This is due to the fact that dates may be incorrect; and if the baby is larger than normal, it may give false fetal ultrasound assessment of gestational age when assessed late in pregnancy.

3. **How accurate are late ultrasounds for establishing gestational age?** Ultrasound after 20 weeks can be inaccurate by 12 days +/− to up to 2.5 weeks at 32+ weeks. Gestational age is determined by measuring one of several fetal skeletal measurements such as biparietal diameter or femur size. These measurements are then used to calculate the age based on a fetal growth percentile chart. Small- or large-for-gestational-age babies will often have incorrect age assessments because of their size.

4. **What is the normal respiratory rate of a neonate at this age?** Respiratory rates for the neonate are normally between 40 to 60 bpm. **How does Baby Cunningham's compare?** With a respiratory rate of 88 to 100 bpm, this baby has tachypnea. **Why do you think this is occurring?** Tachypnea is a compensation measure to increase Baby Cunningham's oxygen levels and clear either a respiratory or metabolic acidosis.

5. **Assess Baby Cunningham's temperature.** The baby is experiencing profound hypothermia. **Is this normal at this age?** Hypothermia is not normal at any age. Although temporary temperature instability may occur right after birth, babies kept in a warm environment and dried immediately should be able to maintain their temperatures. **Why do you think this is occurring?** The environment is cool due to the fact that operating rooms are kept cold to reduce microorganism growth and for the comfort of personnel under layers of clothing. If the preterm infant is chilled, she can lose heat at a rate of up to 0.5 degrees per minute. If the resuscitation equipment is not prewarmed or the oxygen is allowed to flow over the baby or the baby is not properly dried, then the baby can quickly become hypothermic. This hypothermia only increases stress, making the transition to extrauterine life more difficult. This complication is largely preventable. Baby Cunningham is at a higher risk for hypothermia due to her prematurity. Preterm babies lack yellow fat that helps insulate them, preventing heat loss, and brown fat, which is needed to help increase temperature. They lie in an extended posture, which exposes them to greater heat loss.

6. **What is the normal range for neonatal glucose levels?** Most labs will reference 40 to 45 mg for normal newborn glucose as low normal levels with 60 to 80

being normal. **How does Baby Cunningham's compare?** Baby Cunningham is hypoglycemic. **Why do you think this is happening, and what problems could arise if it is not corrected?** Respiratory distress, cold stress, and possible infections all combine to increase the infant's utilization of glucose. This is more critical in a preterm infant with limited glucose stores. Uncorrected hypoglycemia below 40 for more than an hour can cause CNS damage, especially in the preterm infant. When the infant's mother is a diabetic, the fetus may have high insulin levels in order to metabolize the extra glucose he received from the mother. After the birth, the baby (who will maintain a high insulin level for several hours) will quickly metabolize her stored glucose and become hypoglycemic as the increased glucose is no longer being transferred through the cord.

7. **Explain the compensatory principles behind tachypnea, nasal flaring, grunting, and retractions in respiratory distress.** Initially, when infants are not receiving adequate oxygen to the tissues, they will increase their respiratory rate in an attempt to improve oxygenation. This is the easiest compensatory mechanism to be initiated; however, as the infant tires, both the rate and tidal volume will decrease, leading to respiratory failure. If this does not solve the problem, infants will increase the work of breathing by using more force to overcome the increased airway resistance and poor lung compliance in order to increase the airflow. Nasal flaring will result in an attempt to improve air passage and decrease the resistance. If the respiratory distress continues, then expiratory grunting usually begins. This grunting serves to prolong expiratory flow rate by partially closing the glottis, thus creating a positive backpressure. Backpressure helps to maintain expansion by preventing the progressive collapse of the lungs, thus helping to preserve the infant's oxygenation between respirations. It is commonly believed that the severity of the lung disease is related to the loudness of the sounds made with breathing efforts, which is true to a point; but as the infant tires and the respiratory failure progresses, the grunting becomes less apparent and the tidal volume diminishes. Retractions occur when the infant's respiratory effort generates increased negative pressure by using intercostal and assessory muscles to a point where the pressure is much greater in the chest than on the outside. This pressure difference causes the sternum to retract since the chest structure is not well developed in infants, especially preterm ones.

8. **How does the environmental temperature affect Baby Cunningham's chances of survival?** During the initial transition period after birth, infants are vulnerable to temperature instability as a result of exposure to cold environments. Infants must work harder to maintain their temperatures, resulting in increased metabolic rates, increased glucose and oxygen needs, and decreasing surfactant production. All these demands decrease her chance of survival.

9. **Why were cultures done?** Hypothermia, respiratory distress, and hypoglycemia are also signs of a serious neonatal infection. A preterm baby is at a higher risk for infection since his or her immune system is even less developed than that of the term infant. An additional issue for a preterm infant is the lack of antibody transfer that normally occurs in the later stages of the pregnancy. Some of the risk factors for infection are prematurity, low birth weight, premature rupture of membranes, prolonged rupture of membranes, prolonged labor, maternal GBS colonization, maternal genitourinary infection, chorioamnionitis, and meconium stained fluid caused by fetal distress.

10. **How does the APGAR score differ for the preterm infant as opposed to the full-term one?** There is no separate APGAR scoring system for the preterm infant in clinical use. What does differ, however, is the degree to which the preterm infant meets each category. The tone, reflexes, and respiratory status are often very different for the preterm infant and have to be considered. This difference is proportional to the degree of prematurity. When a preterm infant is born, the APGAR assessment is based on what a normal, healthy preterm infant of the same gestational age would have.

11. **How might this situation have been avoided?** The delivery of this preterm baby could have been avoided if labor had not been induced. In normal pregnancies, especially in cases of an uncertain, or inadequately established due date, a baby can be monitored using maternal physical examination, biophysical profiles, and/or NST to avoid prematurity or the development of post-maturity. In this case, the mother was experiencing Braxton Hicks contractions with no cervical changes. If she had been given a sedative, adequate hydration, and encouraged to rest, her contractions would probably have stopped. At a later date when the baby was ready, she would have most likely started labor, progressed normally without the need for induction, and delivered a full-term baby vaginally. If progression failed or fetal distress occurred at that point, then a cesarean section delivery would be appropriate.

12. **What effects related to the parenting process can be expected as a result of the birth complications and infant's condition?** The chances of this mother breastfeeding are greatly reduced in proportion to the period of time it takes to establish the breastfeeding process. Since this infant was admitted to the neonatal intensive care unit, this interrupted contact between parents and child may interfere with bonding.

13. **How can the nurse minimize these consequences?** If Baby Cunningham's mother wishes to breastfeed, it should be encouraged. Breast milk is superior to any formula, and for the preterm baby can be especially beneficial because of the antibodies present. Preterm babies fed only breast milk also have lower risk for necrotizing enterocolitis. The nurse needs to help Baby Cunningham's mother increase ambulation through aggressive pain management, begin to pump her breasts until she is able to nurse the baby, and encourage her to communicate her feelings, fears, and frustration clearly and freely. Referral to a lactation consultant would be very helpful. Bringing the mother to the NICU often, aiding in kangaroo care, and encouraging the family to interact with the baby as much as the baby is able to tolerate are very important for bonding and increase the family's confidence in later caring for the baby.

References

Blackburn, S. (2003). *Maternal, fetal, and neonatal physiology* (2nd ed.). St. Louis, MO: W. B. Saunders Co.

Kramer, M. S, Demissie, K., Platt, R.W., Sauve, R., & Liston, R. (2000). The contribution of mild and moderate preterm birth to infant mortality. *JAMA, 284*(7), 843–849.

Littleton, L., & Engebretson, J. C. (2002). *Maternal, neonatal, and women's health nursing.* Clifton Park, NY: Thomson Delmar Learning.

Rayburn, W. F., & Zhang, J. (2002). Rising rates of labor induction: present concerns and future strategies. *Obstetrics & Gynecology, 100*(1), 164–167.

Case Study 8:   *Baby Long*

1. **During the initial exam the nurse notes that the baby had petechiae on his abdomen and face and also notes that there is some oozing of blood from the venipuncture sites. List possible causes of this finding.**
   - Prematurity
   - DIC secondary to the placenta abruption/sepsis
   - Maternal drug ingestion (heparin, aspirin, quinine, thiazides, and other medications can cause platelet dysfunction in the neonate)
   - Perinatal infection (TORCH or viral)
   - Neonatal infections (Group B strep, herpes, Listeria, Candida, E. coli)
   - PIH/Preeclampsia, HELLP syndrome
   - Maternal antiplatelet IgG based antibodies
   - Placental abnormalities such as placenta abruption and thrombi
   - Decreased platelet production that can occur in some congenital syndromes such as absent radius syndrome and trisomies
   - Asphyxia
   - Platelet function defects as seen in von Willenbrand's disease

2. **The nurse puts a call in to the physician. What initial laboratory studies should the nurse anticipate?** CBC to verify the platelet count and to assess the leukocyte count for any possible infection.

3. **How might results be affected if the nurse decides to collect the blood for these tests by a heel stick?** Heel stick sampling may alter true values of some laboratory tests depending on several factors that may include (1) if the heel was pre-warmed, (2) degree of free blood flow from the puncture site, (3) the amount the heel has to be squeezed in order to obtain a blood sample, and (4) the number of previous lab tests from that same site (since bruising can easily occur with this type of sampling technique). Some of the tests that are affected include the platelet count, hemoglobin, hematocrit, serum CO_2, serum potassium, and some clotting factor tests.

4. **The baby's platelet count is 60,000 units per liter. Assess this finding.** Thrombocytopenia is defined as a platelet count less than 150,000 units per liter with some normal infants as low as 100,000 units per liter in the absence of any disease and without any bleeding tendency. The value of 60,000 units per liter is well below the normal level. At this level there may be spontaneous bleeding following any type of trauma. At the 20,000 to 40,000 units per liter point, spontaneous bleeding can occur, even in the absence of appropriate stimuli. It is not possible to determine etiology from the platelet count.

5. **What would be the next anticipated set of lab tests that might be needed?**
   - Repeat CBC with a manual platelet count but must be drawn centrally in order to eliminate any sampling and indirect testing errors, which may have been present in the original CBC that was drawn from a heel stick. The peripheral smear will allow a direct evaluation of the number, shape, characteristics, and clumping of the platelets that are present.
   - Blood culture as part of the required sepsis workup.

6. **Would the nurse anticipate a spinal tap to be a part of the sepsis workup?** No. This baby is at risk for bleeding due to the low platelet count. A bleed in the spine would be very hard to control and very dangerous.

7. **Should the nurse anticipate the insertion of an umbilical arterial catheter?** Yes. This would be a very good idea since it will eliminate repeated punctures for testing and reduce trauma and opportunities for more bleeding.

8. **What other signs might the nurse note that would be associated with thrombocytopenia?**
    - Generalized superficial petechiae (Clustered petechiae only on the head, face, and upper chest are often normal and occur in response to fetal pressure during vaginal delivery.)
    - Spontaneous bleeding from veinpuncture or mucosal sites
    - Large ecchymoses
    - Muscle hemorrhages

9. **Baby Long was also diagnosed with intravenricular hemorrhage (IVH). What factors contributed directly to this condition?** This is a rare but potentially devastating complication of severe thrombocytopenia, especially in very preterm infants delivered vaginally. While mild IVH is a well-documented complication of the tiny preterm infant, it is an extremely rare occurrence in the term or near-term one. But when IVH does occur as a result of thromboctyopneia, the hemorrhages can be extensive. Recent research has demonstrated reduced risk of IVH if there is a delay in cord cutting in the preterm infant (Mercer, McGrath, Hensman, Silver, & Oh 2003).

10. **List all possible etiologies that are present in the delivery history.**
    - Fetal tachycardia and maternal fever of 101.8° as a potential feature of neonatal sepsis
    - Prematurity
    - Small to moderate placenta abruption (secondary minor trauma to the abdomen following an automobile accident)
    - Maternal disseminated intravascular coagulopathy (DIC)
    - Fetal depression and possible asphyxia based on the low APGARS, especially at 10 minutes.
    - Need for resuscitation at birth

11. **What further lab tests might be included in the evaluation of this thrombocytopenia?**
    - Blood typing in order to look for any ABO or Rh incompatibilities
    - Coombs test to look for the presence of maternal RBC-based antibodies, which may be causing platelet consumption as part of the hemolytic process
    - CBC to assess the possible presence of an infection
    - Coagulation studies including Pt, PTT FSP, INR, CPR, and D-dimer
    - TORCH IgM and IgG titers to look for prenatal infection
    - Blood cultures
    - If persistent, may need maternal antibody studies for antiplatelet antibodies, infant bone marrow studies

12. **What is the treatment that the nurse should anticipate for this infant's thrombocytopenia?**
    - If thrombocytopenia is suspected from prenatal history, then delivery of the infant by cesarean section is done to prevent head trauma and placental injury since these may cause bleeding or accelerate platelet consumption
    - Serial platelet counts can be used to track any trends in the number of circulating platelets

- Maternal corticosteroids prior to delivery may be beneficial in limiting the effects of the maternal antiplatelet antibodies
- Transfusion of maternal and infants ABO/Rh crossmatched platelets if below 20,000 units per liter in full term and 50,000 units per liter in sick or preterm infants without any bleeding and at any level with active bleeding. The baby may need maternal washed platelets for alloimmune thromobocytopenia and exchange transfusion with the immune form if the platelet count does not rise or remain constant after routine platelet transfusion. Remember that between 40 to 60% of the transfused platelets will survive the transfusion
- Infant corticosteroids may help stabilize immune thrombocytopenia and limit the immunity response to the antibodies

References

Bianchi, D. W., Crombleholme, T. M., & D'Alton, M. E. (2000). *Fetology: Diagnosis and management of the fetal patient.* New York: McGraw Hill.

Blackburn, S. (2003). *Maternal, fetal, and neonatal physiology.* Philadelphia: W. B. Saunders Co.

Creasy, R. K., & Resnik, R. (1999). *Maternal fetal medicine* (4th ed.). Philadelphia: W. B. Saunders Co.

Mercer, J. S., McGrath, M. M., Hensman, A., Silver, H., & Oh, W. (2003, September). Immediate and delayed cord clamping in infants born between 24 and 32 weeks: A pilot randomized controlled trial. *Journal of Perinatalogy, 23*(6), 466.

Taeusch, H. W. (2004). *Avery's diseases of the newborn,* (8th ed.). Philadelphia: W. B. Saunders Co.

Part 4: Postpartum Case Studies

Case Study 1: *Molly*

1. **Make a list of possible reasons for Molly's tears.** The most probable cause is normal postpartum blues. Molly, however, may be feeling sad about her birth experience. Her last experience was very satisfying and empowering to her. Although she had an epidural for pain relief, this experience was probably very disappointing to her. Contrary to what many people believe, pain relief is not the major factor in satisfaction of a birth experience. Empowerment is much more significant, and in this birth she felt much more like an object than a person in control. Molly is also probably experiencing perineal pain related to the episiotomy and fourth-degree laceration. She is having greater afterpains since this is her second baby and she is nursing.

2. **What is the relationship between episiotomy and third- and fourth-degree lacerations?** The most common cause of a third- and fourth-degree laceration is the cutting of an episiotomy without proper support of the perineum.

3. **What are the rationales for induction?** Induction is indicated when the mother has gone past her due date (42 weeks gestation) and the baby is showing signs of post maturity. These signs are:
- Reduced amniotic fluid
- Non-reactive non stress test

- Low scores on biophysical profile
- Once membranes are ruptured, presence of meconium in the fluid

Inductions may also be indicated when maternal conditions require an earlier delivery, such as:

- Poorly controlled diabetes
- Severe hypertension
- Eclampsia
- Severe asthma
- HELLP syndrome
- Isoimmunization with high amniotic fluid bilirubin levels
- Renal disease and any other condition that makes continuation of the pregnancy dangerous.

4. **Molly had already experienced a natural birth and was satisfied with her birth. What factors may have caused her to ask for an epidural this time?** Although she did not have medications for her first birth she was in her own home, able to move about and eat and drink as she needed. She was able to determine who would be present and who would not. She could assume any position she felt was comfortable without restriction. She had labor support individuals and was at liberty to tell them what she needed and wanted. These types of empowerment are more effective than medications or epidurals. On the other hand, in the hospital she was not in her own territory, she had no or very little control over her environment, and her movements were restricted due to fetal monitoring and the IV with infusion pump for the induction. She was subjected to noises, smells, and other noxious elements over which she had no control. Pain is intensified in these situations. Pitocin also increases contraction strength quickly. This does not give the woman's body time for endorphins to be released (as usually happens in natural labor) to assist her in dealing with the pain in labor.

5. **What pelvic structures are involved in a fourth-degree laceration?** In addition to mucus membranes, skin, and muscles of the perineum, the anal sphincter is also torn. Finally, there is a tear into the rectal wall.

6. **What special precautions are needed for the woman who has a fourth-degree laceration?** She should not have enemas or suppositories. She will use sitz baths to cleanse the area and promote healing. She will be given stool softeners. Whenever there is a third- or fourth-degree tear, there is always the possibility of later development of fistulas and possible stool incontinence. She will be at a higher risk for infection.

7. **What is the normal amount of blood loss for a vaginal birth?** The normal blood loss is 500 mL.

8. **How does Molly's loss compare?** Anything over 500 mL blood loss in a vaginal delivery is considered postpartum hemorrhage. Molly lost 1000 mL.

9. **List at least two complications that may occur as a result of her postpartum hemorrhage.** Molly will experience fatigue and is at a higher risk of infection. If the bleeding had been more severe, she might have gone into shock or even developed Sheehan's syndrome, which would have interfered with her breastfeeding. (Sheehan's syndrome involves necrosis of the pituitary gland as

a result of the massive hemorrhage, with impaired secretion of one or more of the pituitary hormones). She is also at higher risk for depression.

10. **How should the nurse best approach Molly at this time?** Sit with her for a while. Let her talk about whatever it is she needs to express. If she says she does not know why she is crying, help her to explore her feelings. Tell her that the two things you get in postpartum after the baby is born are sanitary napkins and a box of Kleenex. New moms are expected to use both.

11. **If Molly's older baby wishes to resume breastfeeding, what should she do?** Usually, just letting the older child taste the milk again is enough for the child to feel secure, and he or she does not wish to pursue breastfeeding. If the older child does wish to nurse, and Molly is not against it, it will not cause any harm since she will make as much milk as is demanded of her. She should nurse the youngest baby first, since the infant's only nutrition is the breast milk and the new baby needs the colostrum.

References

Himenick, S. (2003, March). Post ecstatic birth syndrome. *Vital Signs.*

Littleton, L., & Engebretson, J. C. (2002). *Maternal, neonatal, and women's health nursing.* Clifton Park, NY: Thomson Delmar Learning.

Simpson, K. R., & Creehan, P. A. (2001). *AWHONN perinatal nursing* (2nd ed.). Philadelphia: Lippincott, Williams & Wilkins.

Cunningham, F. G., Gant, N., Leveno, K., Gilstrap, L., Hauth, J., & Wendstrom, K. (2001). *Williams Obstetrics* (21st ed.). Norwalk, CT: Appleton & Lange.

Case Study 2: *Candace*

1. **Prior to arriving at the home, what problems does the nurse anticipate at this visit?**
   - Possible cracked, bleeding nipples
   - Possible mastitis
   - Nursing strike
   - Fatigue
   - Postpartum blues

2. **Make a list of the questions that the nurse will ask Candace at the home visit.**
   - Can you show me how the baby acts when you attempt to put him on the right breast? (Observe positioning and baby's reaction.)
   - How long does the baby usually nurse on each side for a feeding? (Does she nurse long enough for the baby to receive the hind milk that will satisfy him and prolong the time before he needs to eat again?)
   - Have you changed your diet in any way since just before this nursing behavior started? (Is she eating something that disagrees with the baby, causing the baby to produce gas and cry? Dairy products eaten by the nursing mother may cause infant colic.)
   - Are you giving the baby a pacifier? (Reduced sucking at the breast due to pacifier use can result in lower milk supply.)
   - Have you used anything on your nipples to clean them or to help with the soreness? (This can cause dryness of the nipples and increase risk of infection.) The baby may also reject the taste.

- Describe your lochia. Have you noticed any foul odor or increases in amount? (Rule out endometrial infection.)
- How much rest/sleep are you getting?
- What have you been eating? (Is she getting adequate nutrition?)
- Are you having any difficulties in voiding? (The nurse needs to rule out UTI.)
- Are you having regular bowel movements? (Constipation can be so disturbing and uncomfortable that it can interfere with a mother's ability to relax and thus feed her baby.)

3. **Make a list of the observations that need to be made at the home visit.**
   - Condition of nipples
   - Condition of breast (Look and feel for hard, red, warm, and painful areas.)
   - Maternal temperature
   - Signs of illness in infant
   - Involution progress of uterus
   - Thyroid gland enlargement; (Rule out postpartum thyroiditis.)
   - Homan's sign (Rule out thrombophlebitis.)

4. **Explain the process of supply and demand as it applies to breastfeeding and milk supply.** The more an infant suckles at the breast, the more milk the mother will produce. Breast milk changes in amount and content as the baby gets older. The consistency of the breast milk and amount of fat content also change throughout a feeding. The hind milk (that milk that is produced at the end of a feeding) is richer and more satisfying. If she was stopping her feedings prior to the baby receiving this hind milk, the baby would not seem satisfied.

5. **Why does it appear to Candace's husband that Candace has lost her milk?** The baby has just reached a point where he is going through a growth spurt. If Candace had been giving him a bottle she just would have increased the amount of milk in the bottle at each feeding. However, breastfeeding requires additional time at the breast suckling for the breast to be stimulated to increase the supply. This is why the baby has been nursing so much for the past day and night. This usually lasts for 24 to 48 hours. Once the supply increases to meet the baby's new needs, he will resume a regular schedule of feeding. Moms need to rest, to drink plenty of fluid, to be very careful about positions to avoid sore nipples, and to feed as the baby demands to increase the supply. They should avoid giving pacifiers and supplemental bottles at this time since both of those will decrease the demand on the breast; thus, there will be less stimulation to produce more milk.

6. **On arrival the nurse finds that Candace's left breast nipple is cracked and bleeding slightly. The nurse also notes that Candace has a fever of 101.2°, seems lethargic, and has an area about the size of a quarter on the underside of her right breast that is firm, painful, red, and warm. Candace tells the nurse that she feels like she has the flu. What is Candace's problem, what probably caused it, and what is the nurse's next action?** This is the typical picture of infectious mastitis. The nurse needs to contact the CNM at the birth center for an antibiotic prescription.

7. **The CNM at the birth center calls in a prescription for ampicillin 500 mg po qid for 10 days. Candace starts crying and asks if this means she can no longer**

breastfeed. **What is the nurse's best response?** On the contrary, she needs to continue to nurse. The antibiotic will not harm the baby, and even if there is a small amount of blood from the nipples, this will not harm the baby. The baby will be getting the mother's own antibodies to protect him from the infection. If the mother were to stop breastfeeding, the milk that remains in the breast will cause an abscess and the problem will get worse, possibly even requiring a surgical incision to drain the abscess. The nurse should suggest she feed the baby on the right breast when the baby is hungriest and then, as he begins to get satisfied, switch to the left side until he is satisfied. To get the baby to take the right breast, hold him in a football hold. This will place the side of his face that he prefers to have next to her the same as if he was on his favorite side (left side). She can take Tylenol for the pain. She should watch the baby for signs of thrush (candidiasis) since antibiotics do cross in a small amount and may allow for the growth of yeast. If the baby develops a yeast infection (thrush), the mother will notice white patches in the baby's mouth that are not easily removed. Eating yogurt with live cultures, or taking live culture acidophilus from the pharmacy, may help reduce her possibility of getting a yeast infection as well as the possibility of the baby getting thrush.

8. **Outline a teaching plan to reduce the possibility of Candace having another mastitis infection.** Mastitis is usually caused from a Staphylococcus infection. Hand washing is essential to reduce this possibility. She should not use soaps on the nipples since that only dries them and makes them more prone to cracking, thus increasing the opportunity for infection to occur. Review proper positioning, latching on, and early signs of hunger with the mother. If she puts the baby to breast when he just begins to show signs of hunger rather than waiting until he is angry, he will not nurse as vigorously and injure her nipples. Review how to remove the baby by breaking the suction with her finger. Review how to support the breast from underneath if she needs to, but not to depress the breast tissue on top of the nipple. Also, be sure that she is comfortable with a variety of positions in order to change the pressure areas on the nipples with each feeding. Reinforce the need to drink to meet her thirst.

9. **Why did the baby only want to nurse on the left side?** This is not unusual and is sometimes called a nursing strike. The baby will often show preferences as to on which side of the mother he likes to have his head. They often prefer the mother's left side. Maybe this is because it puts their head against her heart, a sound they have heard for all of their lives!

10. **How can Candace get him to also nurse on the right side?** To get the baby to take the right breast, hold him in a football hold. This will place the side of his face that he prefers to have next to her, the same as if he was on his favorite side.

11. **Where can the nurse refer Candace for support with her breastfeeding?** Refer her to a local La Leche League leader and/or a lactation consultant. Anticipatory guidance is an essential part of maternity care.

12. **Candace plans to return to work in two weeks. Make a list of decisions and possible problems that she will have to work through during these next two weeks, and after she returns to work, to prepare her and the baby for this transition. Provide alternative suggestions for her to consider.**

- Her mother-in-law is not planning on getting there until she is ready to go back to work. She might consider asking her to come a few days earlier so that everyone can get used to each other (including the baby) before the big day.

- Consider just exactly what she expects from her mother-in-law ahead of time. Does she expect her to do housework as well as care for the baby? If so, is she willing to accept where the mother-in-law will put things, or how she cleans, which may be different from how Candace does things? If this is acceptable, and her mother-in-law agrees, Candace needs to give permission for her mother-in-law to do as she feels comfortable doing.

- Does her mother-in-law agree to the above responsibilities or is she just planning on caring for the baby and expecting the housework to be done by Candace or someone else? This must be clarified ahead of time.

- What is her mother-in-law's philosophy on infant care? Does it match Candace's and her husband's?

- Does the mother-in-law agree with and respect Candace's wishes that the baby will not have anything to eat but breast milk?

- Has she checked at work to see if she will be able to nurse at lunchtime if her mother-in-law brings the baby? Where will she pump her breasts, and where can she store her breast milk? How will she transport it? (Small 6-pack coolers with frozen inserts work very well for short transport times.)

- Is there an infant care facility at work as a backup if needed? Since she is an executive, she may have a private office; can she bring the baby to work with her?

- Where will the baby sleep—in her room, or with her mother-in-law, or in his own room? Who gets up with him at night? If she wishes to continue producing enough milk, she will need to continue to nurse at night.

- How will she get enough rest to meet her home and office responsibilities and still produce adequate breast milk?

References

Biancuzzo, M. (2003). *Breastfeeding the newborn: Clinical strategies for nurses* (2nd ed.). St Louis, MO: Mosby.

Facts for Life: A Communication Challenge, produced for UNICEF, WHO, UNESCO, and UNFPA, rev. ed. 2002.

La Leche League International. (2003). *Leader's handbook* (4th ed.). Schaumburg, IL: La Leche League International.

Littleton, L., & Engebretson, J. C. (2002). *Maternal, neonatal, and women's health nursing.* Clifton Park, NY: Thomson Delmar Learning.

Riordan, J., & Auerbach, K. (2005). *Breast feeding and human lactation* (3rd ed.). Sudbury, MA: Jones and Bartlett.

Case Study 3:   *Juanita*

1. **How might the tension between Juanita's mother and husband, and between Juanita and her mother, be affecting Juanita's breastfeeding?** Juanita may experience difficulties with the process by which the milk is released from the collecting ductules to the baby (letdown or ejection reflex). The letdown reflex is the release of oxytocin from the pituitary in response to infant suckling. The

oxytocin then causes the myoepithelial cells to contract and eject the milk. Women usually feel the letdown as a tingling sensation and can observe the baby swallowing more frequently. Stress is often the cause of failed letdown. If the baby does not get the milk, the baby gets upset, which only adds additional stress.

2. **How might the problem have been avoided?** Knowing ahead of time that there would be a culture conflict, it might have been better if Juanita's mother had come over earlier to give time for the husband and mother to work out some of the expectations. If this was not possible, or Juanita felt that it would not work, then maybe having her mother come over a few weeks later, when her husband had returned to work, would have been better. Her mother could still help her, and her husband would have had an opportunity to establish his routine with the baby first. It is important that couples make very clear what the expectations are ahead of time with any individual who will be helping postpartum.

3. **What suggestions might the nurse give Juanita to relieve the constipation?** The nurse needs to review her diet and if needed offer a stool softener. She was probably discharged with a prescription for one. The nurse can make sure that she is taking them. In some hospitals the mother is given her medications to self-administer during postpartum to get used to taking them prior to going home. The constipation may also be related to the tension in the home. It is also possible that if her mother is now cooking for the family, the change in diet is contributing to her constipation.

4. **How will the nurse assess her breastfeeding problems?** The nurse needs to begin by asking Juanita what problems she was having when she called and asked the nurse to come to the house for a visit. Juanita explains that she only just started to breastfeed the baby this morning. She says that after she got home from the hospital her mother insisted that she not feed the baby the colostrum because it was not good for the baby. She disagreed with her mother but her mother gave the baby a formula anyway, "until the breast milk turns white." Now the baby is having a problem latching on. This delay in feeding and the introduction of a bottle can cause early breastfeeding problems with both latch on and supply and demand. Juanita will need support to get her mother to stop giving the baby formula and encouragement to nurse more often. The nurse can help her with positioning and latch on while she is at the visit.

5. **Are there any community resources that might be helpful for this family?** Juanita might seek support from some of the Cuban women who have been in this country for a few years. They may be able to interest her mother in some outside activities, leaving Juanita and her husband with some time alone with the baby. They may even be able to help her mother understand that young families in this country like to care for their own babies, even the dads. Juanita's mother is more likely to listen to other Cuban grandmothers who are close to her age.

6. **Two days after her delivery, Juanita was given a shot of RhoGAM. At this home visit she asks the nurse why she needed it and if she would have problems with her next pregnancy. How should the nurse reply?** Juanita is Rh negative and the

baby is Rh positive. Her lab work indicated that she did not have antibodies to the Rh-positive factor, and therefore she was given the medication (Rh$_o$ (D) immune globulin (human) is a sterile solution containing IgG anti-D(RH1) for use in preventing Rh immunization) to keep her body from building these. This should protect her for the next pregnancy if she were to have another Rh-positive baby.

7. **Juanita would like to attend a new mothers' group that meets in two weeks. Her mother said that she should not go out for at least 30 days. Juanita is unhappy about this and asks the nurse if she can go. How should the nurse reply?** The nurse can assure Juanita that leaving the house prior to 30 days is not prohibited. She must be sensitive to the cultural difference; however, this is her mother's belief and not Juanita's. The nurse may be able to get the mother to respect her daughter's wishes, although this can be difficult. Respecting another culture does not mean forcing someone to follow it just because they belong to that cultural group, if it goes against their wishes. The nurse can explain that in Cuba there may be less medical care available, and the fear of disease is so high that women avoid being around strangers completely for the first month. By trying to help her understand her mother's viewpoint, Juanita may be able to reason with her mother to accept her wishes. A chance to get out of the home and visit with other new mothers may be very beneficial for Juanita right now.

8. **The nurse does an exam on the infant and notices a safety pin on the baby's undershirt with a religious medal on it. What is the significance of this finding?** This is meant to protect the baby. Many Hispanic families believe in the evil eye, which is a belief that just staring at or overpraising a baby can cause illness. The mother needs to check the safety pin frequently to be certain it does not open. Not only can the open pin injure the baby, but both the pin and medal pose choking hazards.

9. **The baby also has a piece of string in the shape of a circle stuck to her forehead. Juanita looks embarrassed when she sees that the nurse notices the string. What is the significance of the string?** In the Cuban culture a piece of string, wet with saliva and put on the baby's forehead, is used to stop the baby's hiccups.

10. **Juanita tells the nurse that she would like to take a shower and wants to know if it is okay. How should the nurse respond?** Juanita is again questioning her mother's advice. Not bathing or showering for several days after the birth is meant to protect the mother from catching a cold. Once again the nurse can help Juanita try to understand why her mother is concerned, but she can tell her that if she desires there is no medical reason why she should not shower and that good hygiene helps to fight infection. She should remind her not to use soap on her nipples.

Reference

Simpson, K. R., & Creehan, P. A. (2001). *AWHONN perinatal nursing* (2nd ed.). Philadelphia: Lippincott, Williams & Wilkins.

Case Study 4: *Daphne*

1. **Identify at least three questions the nurse should ask Daphne's mother during this initial phone call.**
   - What other symptoms does she have?
   - Does she have a fever?
   - Is she experiencing nausea or vomiting?
   - Does she have any other soreness any place?

2. **Give three possible explanations for Daphne's symptoms.**
   - Postpartum depression
   - Flu
   - Postpartum thyroiditis

3. **The nurse tells Daphne's mother to bring her to the clinic for evaluation. The CNM orders a TSH. Why?** She has many of the symptoms of postpartum thyroiditis. In around 10% of women suffering postpartum depression, thyroiditis is present. In most cases this will resolve on its own. When this condition occurs postpartum, there is a 1 in 4 chance that the mother will develop thyroid disease later.

4. **Which of Daphne's symptoms can be associated with thyroid disease?**
   - Increased appetite with weight loss
   - Headache
   - Moody, agitated, and depressed
   - Fatigue
   - Palpitations
   - Memory loss
   - Concentration impairment
   - Swollen glands may be an enlarged thyroid gland

5. **Her results for her thyroid stimulating hormone (TSH) are 0.24 μIU/mL. What is the most probable diagnosis?** This is borderline low and could mean hyperthyroidism.

6. **What additional test will probably be ordered?** An FT_4 can be ordered. This will confirm or rule out hyperthyroidism.

7. **What are the possible consequences if hyperthyroidism is the problem and it is not diagnosed?** Rarely, women with hyperthyroidism develop thyroid storm, which is a life-threatening condition requiring immediate medical intervention. Individuals with this condition develop exaggerated symptoms of thyrotoxicosis. Occasionally, this condition will develop in women who have not been previously diagnosed with thyroid disease.

8. **Describe the normal involution to be expected for Daphne at this time.** By week three her lochia should be alba, light amount, and without odor; her breasts, since she quit breastfeeding a week ago, may still have milk but any engorgement should be gone.

9. **What are the most common reasons women decide not to breastfeed after they have started?** Reasons why women decide not to breastfeed are sore nipples, unrealistic expectation of how often the baby will feed and sleep, concerns about not having enough milk, embarrassment about feeding in public, and lack of family support.

10. **Daphne states that she is very disappointed that she is not breastfeeding and would like to try to start to breastfeed again. She has bottle-fed for one week now. What is the best response by the nurse?** After hyperthyroidism is ruled out, she can be encouraged to put the baby back on the breast. She will produce enough milk if she is consistent about the nursing. She needs to be taught about positioning the baby to avoid sore nipples in the future. This is called relactation and after only one week should be very easy with adequate stimulation at the breast.

References

Biancuzzo, M. (2003). *Breastfeeding the newborn: Clinical strategies for nurses* (2nd ed.). St. Louis, MO: Mosby.

Riordan, J., & Auerbach, K. (2005). *Breast feeding and human lactation* (3rd ed.). Sudbury, MA: Jones and Bartlett.

Wheeler, L. (2002). *Nurse-midwifery handbook* (2nd ed.). Philadelphia: Lippincott, Williams & Wilkins.

Case Study 5:   *Sueata*

1. **The nurse begins to go over discharge instructions with Sueata. Make a list of the routine discharge instructions given to women who have had normal spontaneous vaginal deliveries.** She needs information about her own care including nutrition and her need for rest. If she has hemorrhoids, she needs instructions on how to reduce them and decrease the pain. The nurse needs to review how to do peri care with her. She needs to know what is normal for lochia flow. She needs to understand how the breasts prepare for milk production, and if she is to bottle-feed, she needs to know now to avoid stimulating the production. She needs to be made aware of signs of infection, including urinary tract infections. For her baby she needs to know the signs of illness and how to bathe and care for her baby. She needs to know about normal newborn checkups, and she needs a copy of the recommended immunization schedule. She must make an appointment for the baby's first follow-up checkup. She needs to be aware of the normal sleep, eating, and elimination patterns for the newborn. She will have to prepare formula and needs to be aware of the dangers of formula contamination, the dangers of propping the baby and how to position the baby for feedings due to increased risk for ear infections when babies take bottles. The nurse needs to review contraception choices with her.

2. **Sueata holds her baby close and cries out, "I hate you. Why couldn't you have been a boy?" How should the nurse respond?** Sueata's nonverbal behavior is in contrast to her words. Her frustrations with having a girl are probably related to the fact that, if she were forced to return to her home country and take the baby, her daughter would face a cruel, hard life. If she is forced to return to her family, they would be more likely to accept a boy than a girl.

3. **Sueata asks about adoption. This is the first time that she has even mentioned that she was thinking about giving her baby up for adoption. How should the nurse approach this subject?** Since Sueata is facing the possibility of going home, she may be having second thoughts about taking a daughter back to that culture and want a better and safer life for her here.

4. **Sueata hands the nurse a letter from the immigration service stating that her student visa will expire in two months. Sueata explains through her tears that if she goes home she will be killed. She has dishonored her family by getting pregnant, and they do not want her back. If she goes home, they may even hire someone to kill her. How likely is it that this story may be true?** This may very well be true. In Pakistan there is such a practice called Karo-Kari. In this practice families can murder with the excuse that the person has dishonored the family. Most of the victims are women. Although the government does not condone the practice, it does little to nothing to stop it or take action against the murderers (Ayazlatif, 2003). Sueata may very well be in danger if she is forced to go back home.

　　Discuss the status of women in the Pakistani culture. Women in Pakistan have no rights. According to Human Rights Watch, when women attempt to report crimes against them, including rape, they often find themselves arrested for adultery. Their testimony is discounted, and if they are ever to be compensated for crimes against them, it is at a much lower rate than it would be for a man in the same situation (Burney, 1999).

5. **What resources might the nurse offer Sueata?** The nurse can make a social service referral, give her the number for Legal Aid to possibly seek counsel on immigration rights, and suggest that she continue her education to be able to extend her student visa. She might check at the college for a counselor who works with foreign students. The nurse may give her information to contact women's rights groups who could also offer legal support and advice.

6. **How is childbearing viewed in the Pakistani culture?** Childbearing and rearing within the arranged family is highly regarded in Pakistan.

7. **Will the baby have United States or Pakistani citizenship?** Because the baby was born in the United States she will have American citizenship. She may also have Pakistani citizenship since Pakistan recognizes dual citizenship.

8. **What methods of birth control might be acceptable to Sueata?** Sueata may feel insulted about being questioned about this topic. She may feel that she made a mistake and does not plan to have intercourse again until she is in a committed married relationship. It is important, however, that the nurse provide her with information about the methods available and how to obtain them.

9. **What specific instructions does she need to care for her breasts since she is not breastfeeding?** She should not stimulate her breasts. This includes no attempts to pump breast milk, she should stand with her back to the shower, and not make love that includes breast caressing. She should wear a snug support bra without underwires 24 hours a day.

10. **Outline information on formula preparation.** She needs to use a formula specifically designed for babies. Milk-based formulas contain approximately 50% more protein than human milk. Although they are processed, they may contain environmental pollutants. Unlike breast milk, they lack the ability to protect the baby from infection. She needs to follow directions on the packaging exactly. Formula prepared with too much or too little water may pose health risks for the infant. Bottled water or boiled tap water may be used. A dishwasher with the temperature set to 120°F will suffice for sterilizing the bottles and nipples. Ready-to-use formula needs no dilution. Powdered formula is mixed using one level scoop of powdered formula with 60 mL (2 oz) of warm water. Concentrate should be mixed with equal parts of the concentrate and water. She should only prepare enough milk in a bottle that the baby usually takes at one feeding. Once the baby has drunk from the bottle, the remaining amount must be disposed of and not stored for the next feeding. Bottles must be kept refrigerated until needed and never heated in a microwave oven. Mothers need to check the temperature prior to giving the formula to the baby. Newborns should be burped after each ounce.

References

Littleton, L., & Engebretson, J. C. (2002). *Maternal, neonatal, and women's health nursing.* Clifton Park, NY: Thomson Delmar Learning.

Ayazlatif, P. (Ed.). (2003). Karo Kari for honour and self pride. *Indus Pak: Resource Center for South Asia and Pakistan.* http://www.31.brinkster.com.

Samya, B. Edited by Regan, E., Brown, R., & Brown, C. (1999). Crime or custom? Violence against women in Pakistan. *Human Rights Watch.* USA.

Case Study 6:   *Roquanda*

1. **Name three common sources of postpartum hemorrhage.** Three common sources are:
   - Uterine atony (May be related to full bladder, hyperstimulation of the uterus in labor, long second stages causing fatigue of the uterine muscles, and/or following Pitocin inductions and augmentations.)
   - Lacerations
   - Hematoma

2. **Compare and contrast them according to the signs and symptoms, precipitating factors, and treatment for each.**

	Uterine Atony/Ineffective Contraction	Lacerations	Hematoma
Signs and symptoms	Boggy uterus often off to the side	Uterus is firm	Uterus is firm
	No birth canal injuries that have not been sutured	Birth canal injuries that may include cervical tears	No birth canal injuries that have not been sutured
	No feelings of pressure	No feelings of pressure	Feelings of pressure; often client complains of need for BM; or pelvic heaviness
	Obvious vaginal bleeding: may be dramatic or slight but constant	Obvious vaginal bleeding: often a steady trickle (however, even with a steady trickle, may hemorrhage to death over several hours)	No obvious blood loss above the normal lochia rubra

(continues)

(continued)

	Uterine Atony/Ineffective Contraction	Lacerations	Hematoma
	VS may indicate shock	VS may indicate shock	VS may indicate shock
			Swelling and discoloration of tissue often, but not always, visible
	Usually no c/o pain	Usually no c/o pain	Pain out of proportion to normal postpartum
Precipitating factors	Use of Pitocin in labor; large baby; long labor; full bladder; placenta accrete; placenta previa; undelivered succenturiate lobe; Duncan delivery of placenta; long second stage	Traumatic (such as shoulder dystocia) and or precipitous delivery; use of episiotomy; use of forceps or vacuum extractor; pushing prior to complete dilatation; bladder status does not affect bleeding	Trauma; forceps and vacuum extractors; large baby and/or OP presentation; prenatal varicosities; coagulation defect; bladder status does not affect bleeding
Treatment	Establish cause. If retained fragments, manual removal is done. If full bladder is interfering, and unable to void, catheterization is done. If simply uncontracted, uterus massage is first tried, then bimanual compression and use of oxytotic type drugs—Hemabate if not asthmatic, Methergine if not hypertensive, and Pitocin mixed in IV or IM (IV push can result in severe hypotension)	Locate the source of trauma by direct visualization and ligate bleeding vessels	Locate hematoma. Vaginal and vulvar are usually seen easily and are self-limiting. Provide volume support and evacuation with surgical closure. Sterile pressure dressings are often used. Vaginal hematomas can be large and will usually result in the complaint of rectal pressure. Incision and evacuation with vaginal pack used to tamponade the edges for 12–18 hours. Retroperitoneal hematoma is the least common. It is the most dangerous. These usually occur in a cesarean section or after rupture of the uterus and require surgery to stop the bleeding

2. **What is the normal expected blood loss for a vaginal delivery?** Up to 500 mL blood loss is normal in a vaginal delivery. Over 1000 mL in a cesarean section is classified as hemorrhage. Most often the loss is underestimated.

3. **Was Roquanda's normal?** Initially, yes. Hers was wnl. However, since she continued to bleed postpartum, she did experience a postpartum hemorrhage. Any woman who is soaking a pad in 30 minutes needs immediate medical attention.

4. **What factors increase the initial blood loss in delivery?** Pitocin use in labor, especially long labors, is associated with postpartum hemorrhage. Since she was being augmented with Pitocin (as opposed to being induced), it is a further indication that her uterus was not contracting well on its own, which should have alerted the staff to her risk. An infant who at term is large for gestational age increases the risk that she may have problems with atony. This is her fourth baby in three and a half years. Closely spaced pregnancies also increase risk of postpartum hemorrhage. Episiotomies always increase blood loss. Trauma from the vacuum extraction may have caused the extension of the episiotomy. Although in itself the vacuum does not cause as much trauma as forceps, it may increase trauma over a normal spontaneous vaginal delivery. Trauma may also cause hematomas.

5. **List four history factors that increase Roquanda's risk for postpartum hemorrhage.**
   - Closely spaced pregnancies
   - Gravida four
   - LGA baby
   - Not breastfeeding

6. **List four labor and delivery factors that increased her risk.**
   - Pitocin use for augmentation
   - Episiotomy
   - Vacuum extraction
   - Long labor and long second stage

7. **Assess her vital signs. Are these normal for postpartum?** No, they are not normal. Postpartum pulse is usually very low. The narrowing of the pulse pressure and low readings are indications of lower blood volume. Her respirations are high.

8. **If not, what is the significance of them?** They indicate shock, especially when accompanied by restlessness.

9. **List at least six other signs of shock related to hypovolemia.** Additional signs of shock are:
   - Air hunger
   - Cool, pale, and clammy skin
   - Decreased or absent urine output
   - Confusion
   - Extreme thirst
   - Decreased pulse pressure
   - Cyanosis
   - Hypothermia

10. **List at least two consequences of postpartum hemorrhage.** She is at risk for:
    - Cardiovascular collapse, shock, and death
    - Increased risk of infection

■ In cases of severe hemorrhage, Sheenan's syndrome may develop with long term effects on her pituitary gland

11. **Why is Roquanda at an even higher risk for problems related to postpartum hemorrhage?** She is Rastafarian, and probably a vegetarian. Also, closely spaced pregnancies have probably left her with iron depletion and iron deficiency anemia, and she is not breastfeeding.

12. **When would you expect Roquanda's hematocrit to be checked? If she had a postpartum hemorrhage, how would you expect it to be reflected in the hematocrit?** Significant changes will not become apparent until 4 hours after the hemorrhage, and complete compensation usually takes about 48 hours. If IV fluids have been given, this may bring about an earlier lowering. Any significant change is important to monitor. A loss of approximately 500 mL will change the hematocrit by 3 percentage points. Women who are otherwise healthy can actually tolerate hematocrits as low as 21% prior to the need for transfusions.

13. **Roquanda's hematocrit is low, and the certified nurse midwife prescribes iron supplements. The nurse is discharging her on her third postpartum day. What information about taking iron supplements needs to be included in teaching Roquanda?** Roquanda needs to know that she should not take her iron supplements with dairy products, tea, or bran. It is best if she can tolerate taking them on an empty stomach. She should also increase her intake of high iron foods and eat these with citrus, such as orange juice.

References

Blackburn, S. (2003). *Maternal, fetal, and neonatal physiology* (2nd ed.). St. Louis, MO: W. B. Saunders Co.

Gabbe, S., Niebyl, J., & Simpson, J. (2003). *Obstetrics: normal & problem pregnancies.* New York: Churchill/Livingstone.

Littleton, L., & Engebretson, J. C. (2002). *Maternal, neonatal, and women's health nursing.* Clifton Park, NY: Thomson Delmar Learning.

Part 5: Well Woman Case Studies

Case Study 1:   *Carina*

1. **Since Carina is underage and does require her mother's consent to have medical care, is it necessary for her mother to be present during the history and physical?** No, it is not necessary for her mother to be present, and since Carina does not wish her to be there, the mother's presence may interfere with Carina's ability to answer and ask questions.

2. **How does Carina's description of her sexual activity impact the manner in which the nurse will pursue the interview?** Carina may be trying to determine the nurse's biases. By asking to be seen without her mother present, Carina may be trying to get information; however, before she opens up to the nurse she is going to "test the waters." She is seeking a comfortable place to expose herself.

3. **Does Carina need a PAP smear and/or STI testing?** Yes. STIs can be spread through oral sex, and Carina's denial does not necessarily mean that she is not having intercourse.

4. **What particular observations will be important for the nurse and the CNM to help determine the cause of her amenorrhea?** Amenorrhea may be primary or secondary. Primary amenorrhea is a condition wherein the woman has never had a menstrual period. Secondary amenorrhea occurs when menstrual periods stop occurring. In this case Carina is being screened for primary amenorrhea. They will look for signs of secondary sexual characteristics: hair pattern growth in the genital area, breast development, development of a maturing body shape. Her body mass index is 17, underweight. This may be very significant. Eating disorders need to be explored.

5. **List five factors that may contribute to the fact that Carina has not yet started her periods.**
   - Is she pregnant?
   - Does she exercise excessively?
   - Is she possibly anorexic, or does she have other eating disorders? (Low BMI and less than 22% fat will interfere with menses.)
   - Does she have excessive body hair (signs of polycystic ovarian syndrome)?
   - What is her stress level?
   - Is her thyroid enlarged?

6. **What possible psychosocial impact might this situation have on Carina?** She may feel inadequate, especially if her friends have all started their menses. She may engage in dangerous sexual activity to compensate for these feelings.

7. **Develop a plan for addressing the abuse situation.** Initially, the nurse/CNM must provide a safe environment for Carina to talk. Depending on Carina's wishes, this may or may not include bringing her mother into the picture. Privacy is very important. Carina must be reassured that anything she shares is confidential, and she must also understand the limits of confidentiality. Carina needs to be made aware that physical abuse is different from passionate love-making and that she is entitled to be safe. She also needs to be aware that abuse usually escalates with time, and although she may not feel that her life is threatened at this time, it could develop into a real threat.

8. **List four questions specifically intended to explore possible abuse that would be appropriate at this visit.**
   - Do you feel that you are safe at home when you are with your boyfriend?
   - Do you ever feel frightened by your boyfriend's behaviors?
   - Do you feel that at times you would like to end your relationship with your boyfriend but don't know how to do it?
   - Do you ever feel forced into sexual activities that you do not want to do?

9. **Outline a teaching plan for Carina.**
   - If her physical exam reveals other signs of secondary sexual characteristics, explain that primary amenorrhea is not unusual for a 15-year-old, and that it is most probable that she will begin her periods within a year.
   - Discuss dangers of STIs, how they are spread, and the consequences to her as a maturing woman, including the effects they can have on her current health and future childbearing, and the life-threatening aspects of AIDS.

- Discuss contraception options.
- Attempt to get her to talk about the abuse by using non-threatening observations and questions. From these responses assess her immediate level of danger. Empower her to say no to whomever it is that is hurting her, and offer her further support if she feels she cannot do this safely. (Parents, counselors, or even police involvement are possible sources.)
- Answer any questions she has regarding her sexuality.

10. Should Carina be offered birth control? Yes. Her responses given here are indicative of someone who is sexually active, and she should be given information on how to prevent an unwanted pregnancy.

Reference

Hawkins, J., et al. (1997). *Protocols for nurse practitioners in gynecologic settings* (6th ed.). New York: The Tiresias Press, Inc.

Case Study 2: *Cyndie*

1. What test should the nurse anticipate? For chlamydia, the antibody, ELISA test Rapid enzyme immunoassay; direct fluorescent antibody tests; DNA probe. The Thayer-Martin smear is considered the "gold standard" for gonorrhea testing. A DNA probe can also be used to check for gonorrhea. A wet mount and whiff test can be used to immediately rule out trichomoniasis, bacterial vaginosis, and yeast infections. She should be advised to be tested for HIV.

2. The client is diagnosed with gonorrhea. What other infection is commonly found with gonorrhea? Chlamydia is commonly found with gonorrhea.

3. Just after her last baby was born Cyndie was diagnosed with gonorrhea/chlamydia infections and treated. How might these infections leave her with secondary infertility? These infections can lead to pelvic inflammatory disease. This disease can scar the fallopian tubes and increase the risk for ectopic pregnancies or cause infertility.

4. Cyndie does not have any drug allergies. What is the most common treatment for these infections? Treatment of choice for chlamydia is azithromycin 1 gm po in a single dose. Doxycycline hydrochloride 100 mg BID for seven days can be used. Ceftriaxone 125 to 250 mg IM or ciprofloxacin 500 mg po single dose can be used to treat the gonorrhea.

5. Should she be re-screened? If so, when? No test of cure is recommended for gonorrhea. If a test of cure (toc) is to be done for chlamydia, then it should be done 3 to 4 weeks after the final dose of medication. If a test of cure is done earlier, the results will indicate a false positive. If she has persistent symptoms after treatment, then she should be reevaluated for re-infection. In these cases partner referral for treatment and education must be addressed. Treatment failure is rare (MMWR, 2002).

6. Is the clinician required to report these diseases to the public health department? If yes, how is this done? Yes, depending on the state health department guidelines. In many states gonorrhea, chancroid, chlamydia, granuloma inguinale, HIV, lymphogranuloma venereum, and syphilis need to be reported. Forms are usually provided through county health departments.

7. **Cyndie also complains of pain around the opening of her vagina on the right side. On inspection the clinician finds an enlarged glandular lump around 2 cm in diameter. This is probably what?** This is most probably an infected Bartholin cyst.

8. **Cyndie also jumps when the clinician moves her cervix. What condition is cervical motion tenderness (chandelier's sign) associated with?** This is associated with inflammation of the fallopian tubes. It is seen in ruptured tubal pregnancies and in pelvic inflammatory disease (PID) where the tubes are infected.

9. **Outline the teaching the nurse needs to provide to Cyndie prior to her leaving the office today.** The nurse needs to instruct her to avoid sexual intercourse until therapy is completed and until she and her sex partner(s) no longer have symptoms. She should use condoms until after she has finished the full treatment. She should stay out of the sun if she is given doxycycline. She should return to the clinic if symptoms return.

10. **If Cyndie were pregnant, how would her treatment be different?** She could still be treated with azithromycin 1 gm po in a single dose and Rocephin. These are pregnancy category B drugs.

References

MMWR. (2002). http://www.cdc.gov/std/treatment/default.htm.

Varney, H., Kriebs, J., & Gegor, C. (2004). *Varney's midwifery* (4th ed.). Sudbury, MA: Jones & Bartlett.

Case Study 3:   *Anna*

1. **What is the significance of the fact that Anna breastfed all of her children for at least a year each?** Breastfeeding for at least six months reduces the chances of developing breast cancer during the pre-menopausal years.

2. **What screening and/or diagnostic tests are appropriate for Anna at this visit?**
   - PAP
   - STI screen, including HIV screen
   - Mammogram
   - Cholesterol screen
   - Thyroid screen
   - CBC
   - Her immunization should be reviewed and updated if needed.
   - She should have a TB screen done. (Miami is an urban area with a highly mobile international population that is known to have a high exposure to tuberculosis. Yearly PPD screening is recommended for the general population, and PPD every six months for health care workers is recommended.)

3. **Anna describes the lump as very small, having irregular edges and not feeling painful. What type of lump commonly presents with these characteristics?** These are non-reassuring signs more commonly associated with a malignant cancer.

4. **The nurse examines Anna and finds the lump is fixed and located in the upper outer quadrant of the breast. Are these additional findings reassuring or non-reassuring?** These are also non-reassuring and are often associated with malignant cancer.

5. **The nurse also notices no scaling or nipple discharge and no infraclavicular or supraclavicular adenopathy. However, she did note edema in the auxiliary area of Anna's right arm. What is the significance of this?** If scaling on the nipple had been present, it could have meant Paget's disease, which is a serious form of breast cancer. Nipple discharge is usually either a hormone imbalance or an infection. Edema in the auxiliary area may be a problem related to impaired lymph drainage.

6. **Which diagnostic test is most appropriate to start with for Anna—an ultrasound or a mammogram?** A clinically palpable mass needs to be assessed with a mammogram as the first examination. The mammogram will help to distinguish between a solid and a fluid-filled mass. A woman in her teens or twenties who is having a screening examination (without palpable masses) is often examined first by ultrasound due to the fact that the breast tissue is more dense in the younger years.

7. **If the mammogram reveals a suspicious lump, what will be the next step to diagnosis if it is cancer?** The next step will be a needle biopsy or regular biopsy and lumpectomy with the possibility of further tissue removal if the biopsy is malignant. This will probably be followed with chemotherapy and/or radiation.

8. **Give at least two possible causes of Anna's fatigue that are not related to the breast lump.**
   - Anna is very busy and may just not be getting enough rest
   - Possible hypothyroidism
   - Possible anemia
   - Stress may also cause fatigue
   - Infection increases fatigue

9. **List at least three questions that the nurse needs to ask Anna to help determine the cause of her fatigue.**
   - How much sleep do you get?
   - What are your periods like?
   - What you eat in an average day?
   - What is a typical day like for you?
   - How much stress would you say that you experience?
   - How long have you felt this fatigue?
   - Have you experienced fever or night sweats?

10. **Identify community resources that can offer support to Anna and her family if the breast lump is cancerous.** At http://www.nabco.org the National Alliance of Breast Cancer Organizations provides a great site for finding community resources.

11. **Are Black women more or less at risk for breast cancer?** Although the risk for developing breast cancer is not higher in Black women, the risk of dying from it is greater. This may be due to the fact that Black women are less likely to have

access to regular preventative care than non-Black women. Often, when cancer is discovered, the breast cancer is more advanced. Risk factors that are significant are age over 50; being a female; a personal history of breast, ovarian, or endometrial cancers; and a positive family history of breast cancer. Other risk factors are delayed childbirth to after 30 for a first completed pregnancy, not ever having breastfed for at least six months, early menarche, late menopause, exposure to ionizing radiation; nulliparity, and exposure to hormone therapy, including estrogen-containing birth control pills and hormone replacement therapy. Other possible factors include obesity, diets high in fat, high alcohol intake, environmental exposure to such things as pesticides, and smoking.

References

HHS Affirms value of mammogram for detection of breast cancer. (2002). HHS Release, U.S. Dept. of Health and Human Services.

Littleton, L., & Engbretson, J. (2002). *Maternal, neonatal and women's health nursing.* Clifton Park, NY: Thomson Delmar Learning.

Morgan, G., & Hamilton, C. (2003). *Practice guidelines for obstetrics and gynecology* (2nd ed.). Philadelphia: Lippincott, Williams & Wilkins.

Case Study 4: *Jodi*

1. **Discuss HPV infections.** Condylomata acuminata is a sexually transmitted illness caused by the human papillomavirus (HPV). It is possible that it can be transmitted through fomites. If the disease is not active, it cannot be passed. It cannot be cured. HPV does not always cause a visible lesion. Subclinical infections can occur on the cervix as well as externally. The HPV virus can be manifested in several different ways such as venereal warts, intraepithelial neoplasia, and squamous/epithelial carcinoma. There are more than 80 types of the HPV virus. The HPV types 6, 11, 16, 18, 31, 33, 35, and 39, among others, have been associated with cervical and vulvar cancer. This is a very common infection with estimates of from 10% to 50% of sexually active women being positive for the infection. Initial infection rates are highest in young women, usually occurring shortly after the onset of sexual activity. Ninety-eight to ninety-nine percent of all cervical cancers are HPV positive. The incubation period is from two weeks to nine months, or possibly even years.

2. **If a client complains of discomfort associated with the HPV treatment, what suggestions can the nurse give her for pain relief?** At the time of treatment a dusting of baby powder onto the affected area and 2.5% Nupercainal ointment on the area may be helpful. Afterward, try warm or cool sitz baths several times a day and two Tylenol tablets every 4 to 6 hours. She should be advised to keep the area clean and dry. She may use a hair dryer on low setting. If she wears underpants, they should be cotton and changed often.

3. **How should the nurse respond to Jodi's question about the swimming pool?** HPV infections may very rarely be transmitted by fomites. It is, however, very unlikely that this is the source of her infection; direct person-to-person sexual contact is the usual form of transmission. Chlamydia and gonorrhea are not transmitted by fomites.

4. **Since these PAP smears are coming back abnormal, what treatment should the nurse anticipate that Jodi will be referred for?** When reading the results of a PAP screen, the nurse will find three parts. The first part is a statement of adequacy. This tells the clinician if the specimen that was received by the lab was adequate for testing. The second part is a statement that says the sample is either normal or abnormal. If the sample is found to be abnormal, a further distinction will be made. It may be benign cellular changes (infections or changes associated with reparative processes such as childbirth and certain gynecologic procedures). Benign cellular changes do not progress to cancer. These are usually classified as atypical squamous cells of undetermined significance (ASCUS). It is the most common type of abnormal result. It is not cancer. Many times these resolve on their own. Most women will be retested in a few months. High-risk women will have colposcopy right away. The infections may be either sexually transmitted or non–sexually transmitted. Examples of sexually transmitted infections are Trichomonas vaginalis, syphilis, chlamydia, gonorrhea, and herpes simplex. For these infections, the woman and her partner require treatment. Other infections are not necessarily sexually transmitted. They are caused by fungal organisms morphologically consistent with Candida and bacterial vaginosis (BV). These conditions are usually related to a change in the normal flora of the vagina. Systemic antibiotic use can increase vaginal fungal infections. Douching destroys the normal lactobacilius in the vagina and can increase risk for bacterial vaginosis. Benign cellular changes may be inflammation; atrophy with inflammation, usually seen in post-menopausal women; following radiation; and sometimes seen when women have intrauterine contraceptive devices (IUD).

Abnormal changes that require further investigation are classified as epithelial cell abnormalities, which are not necessarily cancer at this time but may be or may lead to cancer. These are either squamous cell or glandular changes. This finding needs a retest in three months. Squamous intraepithelial lesion (SIL) may be either low-grade (LSIL) or high-grade (HSIL) squamous intraepithelial lesion. The LSIL may be due to cellular changes associated with human papillomavirus They require a colposcopy within four weeks. These have mild dysplasia. The high-grade squamous intraepithelial lesion (HSIL) requires a colposcopy immediately. These may be moderate dysplasia (CIN-II) but still not cancer. Severe dysplasia and carcinoma in situ (CIN-III) is cancer but is limited to the cervix and still has an excellent chance of cure. When glandular cells are present, they are usually endometrial cells not usually found in the PAP test. This finding is called atypical glandular cells of undetermined significance (AGCUS). This could indicate cervical or endometrial problems. This finding is usually followed with endocervical curettage and endometrial biopsy.

Finally, a PAP report will contain a hormone evaluation. This evaluation looks at the hormonal pattern and determines if it is consistent with the woman's age.

The treatment ranges from repeating the PAP (which is done for the inflammatory type of changes) to colposcopy, biopsy, and some type of cervical conization, all the way to complete hysterectomy for the CIS or squamous cancer changes. Cervical conization consists of either the hot wire loop (LEEP), cold knife (CKC), cryotherapy, or surgical excision.

In this case, the first PAP smear with ASCUS was treated appropriately but the follow-up should have been repeat PAP every six months until she had three normal PAP results. Once the PAP smear became abnormal again, with HPV changes, a cervical conization should have been done during her early pregnancy. Now that the PAP smear is HGSIL, aggressive full cervical conization with wide excision must be done or, since she is planning on no further children, a complete hysterectomy.

5. **What is the significance of the different grades of different PAP smear abnormalities?** The higher the degree of abnormal cellular growth, the higher the cancer risks, which are as high as 15 to 25% for HGSIL dysplasia. The inflammatory changes are often secondary to various types of vaginal infections and only require close follow-up after the infection is treated. When vaginal discharge is noted at the time of the PAP, the best management would be to do a wet mount and treat the vaginal infection, then do the PAP after 6 to 8 weeks when the vaginal infection has been cleared. This can eliminate the need for many colposcopies since once the infection is cleared up the PAP will usually come back normal. At the early stages, with either atypia-favoring HPV or mild to moderate dysplasia, a colposcopy is required. With higher levels of dysplasia or cancer in situ, aggressive conization or hysterectomy is needed. The woman needs close follow-up for at least two years of normal examinations and even more in the presence of an additional risk factor such as HPV infection reoccurrence or a family history of gynecological cancer.

6. **What is the significance of and treatment for gonorrhea and chlamydia?** Gonorrhea and chlamydia often occur together, and when one is diagnosed it is often wise to treat for both. These two infections are the most common causes of pelvic inflammatory disease, leading to tubal scarring and possible ectopic pregnancies. With the exception of HPV, most of the other sexually transmitted infections only cause inflammation on the PAP smear, which corresponds to inflammation without atypia or ASCUS. The preferred treatment for chlamydia is azithromycin, doxycycline with erythromycin, or ofloxicin as secondary alternatives. The gonococcus organism is best treated with ceftriaxone with cefotaxime, spectinomycin, or Ciprofloxacin as secondary treatments. Penicillin is no longer an option because of the drug resistance that has developed in most gonococcus strains. Another common sexually transmitted infection that is known to cause abnormal PAP smears and is also associated with preterm labor is Trichomonas vaginalis. It is treated with metronidazole (Flagyl) po, but not during the first trimester of pregnancy because of the possible teratogenic effects on the fetus.

7. **Jodi says she is tired of using birth control and asks the nurse about permanent sterilization. How should the nurse reply?** Because some women who choose sterilization regret the decision later, it is important to emphasize the fact that this is permanent and should not be done with the plan to reverse it later on. Since she is only 31 years old, she should take her time in making this decision. If she changes her mind later, reversing a tubal ligation is difficult and often impossible. Part of the consent will be a full explanation of the many good contraceptive alternatives that are available to her. The nurse also needs to consider the final cervical biopsy results. If after repeat aggressive conization the PAP smears or cervical biopsy continue to show HGSIL, either squamous cell cancer or adenocarcinoma, then hysterectomy may be the best choice. The clinician will discuss these with her, and the nurse can follow up by answering her questions that may come up following the counseling.

8. **What are the clinical consequences of a premature surgical hysterectomy?** The performance of a complete hysterectomy may or may not cause premature surgical menopause. A complete hysterectomy does not routinely include the removal of the ovaries, which is called an oophorectomy. Even if the ovaries are left, if they have been dependent upon the uterine artery for blood flow, they may atrophy and even fail if this blood flow is disrupted by the hysterectomy (disruption of uterine artery blood flow).

When menopause occurs the woman may experience dyspareunia, urinary stress incontinence, body hair changes, vasomotor changes, diaphoresis, subtle breast changes, emotional irritably, tension headaches, and mild depression. Some of the internal bodily changes include an acceleration of coronary artery disease and the loss of bone mass or osteoporosis. The severity of symptoms is variable from person to person. The woman's personal attitude about menopause and her feelings about the loss of reproductive function as well as the physical factors such as the amount of body fat, life-long duration of estrogen exposure, the age and speed of ovarian failure onset, baseline health status, level of physical conditioning, nutritional habits, smoking, and alcohol intake will all determine her adjustment postoperatively. The average age for the onset of menopause in the United States is 51 years, but individually it is often similar to that of her own mother. For years women have been prescribed hormone replacement therapy (HRT) with the mistaken belief that it was harmless and promoted better postmenopausal health. The basic risk factors include a personal or family history of either estrogen-sensitive breast or endometrial cancer, previous thromboembolism, age greater than 45, and heavy smoking. Fortunately, cervical cancer types are usually not hormone receptor positive. However, breast cancers are often hormone receptor positive. HRT does not prevent or reduce coronary artery disease or stroke. Coronary artery disease may actually be accelerated over the first five-year period of therapy with HRT. Osteoporosis is only slowed during the time that the woman is actually taking the HRT. Within a short time after discontinuing HRT her risks are the same as if she had never taken it. There are other options to reduce risk from osteoporosis such as alendronate (Fosamax) and raloxifen (Evista) for treatment and prevention. In cases where HRT is contraindicated Depo-Provera or clonidine can be used for hot flashes and selective serotonin reuptake inhibitors (SSRI) for mood instability. Natural progesterone has been shown to reduce risk and even promote new bone growth. It is available without prescription and does not carry the health risk of the artificial progesterone (Progestin). Natural progesterone often reduces other menopausal symptoms as well. Women around the world have taken Black cohosh for years for menopausal symptoms with very positive results. Nonpharmacological measures for menopausal symptoms include exercise, balanced diet, Vitamins E and B complex, adequate calcium intake, and avoidance of caffeine, smoking, and alcohol. As a side note for those women who have undergone natural menopause without any hysterectomy and wish to take HRT, they must take the progestin/estrogen combination to reduce risk of estrogen-stimulated endometrial cancer.

9. **What are the different treatment options available for these types of cutaneous lesions?** The treatment of HPV-related cutaneous lesions require lesion destruction. This destruction can be done either surgically or pharmacologically. The surgical procedures include any of the following: cryotherapy, laser,

surgical excision, or electrosurgery. Some of the pharmacological options consist of trichloroacetic acid (TCA), podophyllin, and 5-FU or imiquimod cream.

10. **What type of continuing patient instructions and follow-up will be needed?** The client needs to check herself with a mirror frequently to look for new warts. She needs PAP smears from every three to six months until she has had three normal PAP results.

11. **Will the partner need to be treated for any of the infections?** Yes. The partner needs to have aggressive treatment for all of these STIs that have complicated this problem because they will reoccur if they are not treated.

References

Bethesda 2001 Terminology. www.bethesda2001.cancer.gov.

Choma, K. (2003). ASC-US and HPV testing. *American Journal of Nursing, 103*(2), 42–50.

Morgan, G., & Hamilton, C. (2003). *Practice guidelines for obstetrics and gynecology.* Philadelphia: Lippincott, Williams & Wilkins.

CDCP 2002. *STD treatment guidelines.* www.cdc.gov.

Case Study 5:   *Jing*

1. **What is endometriosis, and how does it affect the health of the women who develop the disorder?** Endometriosis is the abnormal growth of endometrial tissue outside of the uterus. Because it is often asymptomatic, it is hard to state how frequently it occurs. Some estimates are that it occurs in 10 to 15% of women. This tissue responds to the cyclic hormones and bleeds during periods of the menses. This tissue may be found in many locations throughout the pelvis, abdomen, and distant sites such as the brain, spinal cord, lungs, and heart. These areas become larger, more consolidated, and better formed with each passing cycle.

2. **What are the classic signs and symptoms?** Pain is not always in proportion to the amount of endometriosis present. The classic symptoms include dysmenorrhea, dyspareunia, irregular menses, premenstrual bleeding, cyclic hematuria, painful defection, and chronic pelvic pain associated with or just prior to menses. Over a period of time this repeated bleeding stimulates formation of scar tissue and adhesions, which immobilize and may strangulate abdominal and pelvic structures. This causes pain and infertility. Pain also comes from the enlarged uterus and its increased dysfunctional bleeding that sometimes is associated with endometriosis. Premenstrual diarrhea may indicate rectosigmoid endometriosis.

3. **What is the natural course of endometriosis?** There are several theories about the development of endometriosis. One theory states that an excessive proliferation of endometrium refluxes though the fallopian tube(s) out into the adenxa first, then later into the pelvis. This is called retrograde menstruation. Other theories blame the lymphatic system for spreading the endometrial tissue. There are some theories that cite the immune system as having a role in the origin of endometriosis. A decreased immune response has been found in women with endometriosis. Another theory discusses the possibility of undifferentiated cells of the peritoneum undergoing changes under hormonal

influences and becoming endometrial cells outside the uterus. This is called the theory of coelomic metaplasia. The displaced endometrial tissue implants begin to enlarge and spread under the continuing estrogen influence from each passing menses. Tissue may also spread during gynecological surgery, lymphatic, or vascular metastasis. Each menses then continues the spread and further development of adhesions. Distortion of the fallopian tubes may cause infertility, or if conception does occur, it may cause ectopic pregnancy. Depending on the place that the endometrial tissue implants, the symptoms will vary. On the bladder it can cause dysuria, polyuria, and cyclic hematuria. Lesions on either the colon or the small bowel will lead to the symptoms of abdominal cramps, nausea, diarrhea, and pain on defecation. Endometrial tissue in the cul-de-sac is especially painful. Adhesions from endometriosis can cause bowel obstruction. If left untreated, the woman will develop an acute abdomen requiring immediate surgery.

4. **What are the different risk factors for the development of endometriosis?** Risk factors that have been associated with the development of endometriosis include a history of early onset of menses, frequent menses of less than 28 days, long periods (over 7 days), small cervical os that has not been previously dilated, delayed childbirth, thin and tall stature, one dominant fallopian tube that is larger than the other one, and any kind of Müllerian abnormalities. There is some evidence that supports a familial tendency. Other more controversial factors include socioeconomic status, and minor racial difference with the incidence in Asian and White women slightly higher than in Black or Hispanic women. Some personality traits have been mildly correlated with the development of endometriosis, such as being overly anxious, a perfectionist, overachiever, or excessively underweight secondary to eating disorder. The risk decreases when the amount of menstrual flow is curtailed or decreased such as in excessive exercise, in grand multiparas, and in those who have used low-dose birth control pills for long periods of time.

5. **What are the different treatment options available for endometriosis?** The treatment of endometriosis is determined by the woman's desire to get pregnant and her symptoms. Pharmacologic suppression of endometriosis can be achieved with hormonal regulation. The hormones are manipulated to mimic a time period when menstrual changes do not occur, such as in pregnancy or menopause. Continuous or cyclic oral contraceptives may be prescribed. Progestins (medroxyprogesterone acetate 30 mg/day) can be used alone in situations where estrogens are contraindicated. GnRH agonists (nafarelin, Lupron, Zoladrex) can be used to bring about amenorrhea and provide pain relief and resolution of the active disease. Side effects of GnRH agonists also mimic menopause. Surgical therapy is required when an adnexal mass or endometrioma is present and has to be removed or when the client is suffering very painful episodes. Smaller lesions can be destroyed with laser either at the time of laprotomy or through less invasive laproscopy. In addition to surgery, the pain can be managed with analgesics. If the woman wishes to become pregnant and the endometriosis has caused infertility, she may need reconstruction surgery to remove adhesions and correct distortion of the fallopian tubes.

In vitro fertilization (IVF) and gamete intrafallopian transfer (GIFT) are other options for attaining a pregnancy. GIFT involves a laparoscopy and usually general anesthesia. Several mature eggs and 50,000 sperm are deposited into the mother's fallopian tubes. This allows for fertilization and early embryonic development to take place in the natural environment of the fallopian tubes.

During early days of IVF, the GIFT method had a much higher rate of pregnancies achieved. However, recently IVF successes approach those of the GIFT procedure. For the IVF method, ova maturation is stimulated for retrieval and use by using gonadotropins in combination with gonadotropin releasing hormone (GnRH) agonist to optimize follicular development. GnRH agonists, Lupron and Synarel, produce an initial increase in the endogenous FSH and LH release from the pituitary gland. This may last several days. Both of these drugs are able to suppress the gonadotropins release as long as the medication is adequately administered. Gonadotropins are administered at the same time as the GnRH agonists. Exogenous follicle stimulating hormone (FSH) then promotes ovarian follicular development and egg maturation (despite GnRH agonist suppression of endogenous FSH). This is important because it limits subsequent ovarian follicular development. In some cases clomiphene citrate is used (with or without gonadotropins) to stimulate ova maturation; however, multiple pregnancy, ovarian hyperstimulation syndrome, ovarian torsion, and possibly ovarian epithelial carcinoma may result from clomiphene citrate (Clomid) use. IVF procedures are very expensive, costing from $5000 to $10,000 each time they are attempted. Only about one-quarter of the attempts result in viable pregnancies.

Ethical concerns may arise, depending on the religious and moral convictions of the parents, if multiple ova are produced and fertilized, jeopardizing the mother's ability to carry the pregnancies to viability without destroying some of the developing embryos/fetuses. This may cause conflict for Jing because the Shinto religion teaches respect for all life.

6. **What are chocolate cysts, and how are they treated?** Chocolate cysts, or endometriomas, primarily develop on the ovary and in the pelvis. These occur when the ectopic endometriosis lesions become large and necrotic and hemorrhage into the center of the cyst. The enlarged cyst can become very painful. When these cysts burst, they may mimic pyelonephritis, acute appendicitis, or ectopic-tubal pregnancy. The name "chocolate cyst" refers to the dark brown, non-coagulating thick blood that fills the cyst. These cysts are classic findings in endometriosis. If they occur on the ovary, they can lead to painful ovulation. This type of cyst rarely resolves spontaneously and usually ruptures, spilling its contents into the peritoneum and causing severe abdominal pain.

7. **Does endometriosis cause cancer?** While the occurrence of malignancy arising from endometriosis is rare, it has occurred. The site is almost exclusively ovarian, and the transition is to either clear cell or endometrial carcinoma. It has been noted that up to 4% of all endometrial lesions have epithelial atypia, which in turn is a high-risk factor for developing epithelial malignancies of the pelvis. Studies have been limited on this subject.

8. **Identify several resources that the nurse can refer Jing to for support.** There are good sources that the nurse can give to Jing to learn more about her condition and obtain support. These are the Endometriosis Association at http://www.endometrosisassn.org, the American College of Obstetricians and Gynecologists at http://www.acog.org and the Endometrosis Research Center at http://www.endocenter.org.

9. **Describe how endometriosis is staged.** The American Society of Reproductive Medicine staging system is based on the depth, location, and size of the endometriotic implants; presence or absence of cul-de-sac obliteration; and the extent of the adhesions. Symptoms have no bearing on the staging.

10. **Are there any natural treatments that have been successful in reducing pain from endometriosis?** Dietary changes may help some women with mild symptoms. Other alternative therapies that have been helpful are natural progesterone and acupuncture. According to Christiane Northrup (*Women's Bodies, Women's Wisdom*, 1998) natural progesterone helps counteract endometriosis by decreasing the effects of estrogen on the endometrial lesions. It is free of side effects.

References

Daiter, E. (2004). *Infertility tutorials.* Coastal Publications, LLC. http://www.infertilitytutorials.com/index.cfm.

Northrup, C. (1998). *Women's bodies, women's wisdom.* New York: Bantam Books.

Sills, E. S., Perole, M., Stamm, L. J., Kaplan, C. R., & Tucker, M. J. (2004). Medical and psychological management of recurrent abortion, history of postneonatal deaths, ectopic pregnancy and infertility: successful implementation of IVF for multifactorial reproductive dysfunction. A case report. *Clinical & Experimental Obstetrics & Gynecology 31*(2):143–146.

Case Study 6:

Sylvia

1. **Identify at least three possible reasons for Sylvia's weight gain.** She may have become more sedentary since her stroke. As women get older they will often undergo a slight decrease in metabolism, which causes them to gain a few extra pounds. Weight gained around the "middle" is more critical to overall health than overall weight gain. This is associated with increased risk for heart attack. Possible hypothyroidism may account for the weight gain. She is showing other symptoms of this problem. Finally, many individuals will eat more when they are depressed, and this could account for her weight gain.

2. **Make a list of the lab tests that the nurse should anticipate will be ordered for Sylvia at this visit.** She will need a complete blood count; FOBT x3 (hemocult) to screen for colorectal cancer; TSH with reflex T4. She needs a cholesterol screen, bone density scan, a mammogram, and a PAP smear.

3. **Give four possible causes for her fatigue.** Her fatigue may be related to anemia from the heavier periods, stress related to her job, increased responsibilities of caring for her mother, depression, and/or hypothyroidism.

4. **Sylvia has yearly mammograms, does breast self-exams, gets a yearly complete physical, and has no family history of cancer. Using the data from her profile and the case study, assess her risks for breast cancer.** Although having routine exams increases the likelihood that if she develops breast cancer it will be discovered earlier, it does not reduce her risks for developing breast cancer. Smoking and alcohol intake increase her risk. A unilateral blackish-green discharge is possibly a sign of infection. A culture should be obtained as well as cytologic studies.

5. **How does Sylvia's lifestyle contribute to her chances of having another stroke?** Sylvia has a family history of stroke (her mother). She has had a stroke herself,

she continues to smoke, and she lives a high-stress life. Her cholesterol levels need to be reviewed as well as her diet. Her history of hypertension and previous stroke contribute to her risk for a repeat stroke as well as other cardiovascular diseases.

6. **How common is thyroid disease in women?** Thyroid disease is very common in women, especially in peri- and postmenopausal women. According to the American Association of Clinical Endocrinologists, women are five to eight times more likely than men to suffer from thyroid disease. Incidence of hypothyroidism (underactive thyroid) increases with age, with peak onset occurring between the ages of 35 and 60 (AACE, 2001).

7. **Assess her risks for cardiovascular disease.** She is Black American and smokes two packs a day. Her LDL is high, and she has hypertension. She is overweight, lives a high-stress lifestyle, and has a history of depression. She also has a history of stroke. She is at very high risk for a heart attack and/or another stroke.

8. **Assess her menstrual changes.** These are typical perimenopausal changes. As estrogen continues to build the endometrial base without progesterone withdrawal, the endometrial lining grows until it can no longer be supported. The result is the shedding of the lining in a disorganized irregular manner. Her thyroid dysfunction and stressful lifestyle may also contribute to this condition. Fibroids may also make it worse. She may develop anemia as a result of this repeated heavy blood loss.

9. **Analyze the following lab results:**
   LDL 146 mg/dL   high
   VLDL 41 mg/dL   high
   HDL 33 mg/dL   low
   Triglycerides 207 mg/dL   high
   Total cholesterol 220 mg/dL   Her total cholesterol is over the highest acceptable level. Her ratio of LDL to HDL is 6.67. Ideally, it should be 3.4 to 1 and acceptable levels of 4.5 to 1 in women. She needs to bring down her VLDL and LDL and raise her HDL. Diet, exercise, and possibly lipid-lowering drugs may be needed.
   TSH 10.2 μIU/mL   She will need a follow-up with a serum-free T$_4$ (FT$_4$). Her thyroid stimulating hormone is high, indicating a need to further test for hypothyroidism. She also has an enlarged thyroid gland, a bruit, and a disordered menstrual pattern. This supports a diagnosis of hypothyroidism.

10. **Sylvia is a Black American woman. How might her race impact on her health risk factors?** Silvia is exhibiting several conditions that are more prevalent in the Black population. Hypertension, fibroids, obesity, and stroke are all more prevalent in the Black population.

11. **Many women will self-medicate with over-the-counter medications, herbals, etc. Review her prescription medications and her self-medication and comment on any interactions she needs to be made aware of.** The calcium taken at the same time as the atenolol will decrease the effects of the atenolol. This may be a reason why her hypertension is not responding to the therapy. Taking the calcium is a sound idea; however, she needs to be advised not to take it within six hours of the atenolol. If after she makes this change in the timing of her medications

her hypertension does not respond to the atenolol, she should be prescribed diuretics. The St. John's wort will interfere with her fluoxetine (Prozac) with the result being more depression. She should take either the fluoxetine or the St. John's wort, not both. Sylvia needs to be referred back to her primary clinician for further evaluation of her thyroid and hypertension symptoms.

References

Overweight prevalence. (2000). http://www.cdc.gov/nchs/fastats/overwt.htm.

Wheeler, L. (2002). *Nurse-midwifery handbook* (2nd ed.). Philadelphia: Lippincott, Williams & Wilkins.

Whitneye, N., Cataldo, C. B., & Rolfer, S. R. (2002). *Understanding normal and clinical nutrition.* Belmont, CA: Thompson/Wadsworth Learning.

Thyroid through the ages: Midlife (menopause). http://www.aace.com/pub/tam2001/tam-midlife.php.

Risk factors. http://www.nuff.org/health_riskfactors.htm.

JNC-VII report on management of hypertension. http://hp2010.nhlbihin.net.

Case Study 7: **Josephine**

1. **Identify at least three health risks for Josephine and give at least two pieces of supporting data for each of your choices.**

   Risk: Osteoporosis
   Supporting data:
   Smoked for 20 years
   Underweight (BMI 18.3)
   White
   Poor nutrition
   Sedentary lifestyle
   Decreased height
   Backache

   Risk: Heart disease
   Supporting data:
   Age
   Family history (mother)
   Smoked for 20 years
   Surgical menopause
   Sedentary lifestyle

   Risk: Breast cancer
   Supporting data:
   First-degree relative with breast cancer
   Age
   Smoked for 20 years
   HRT for five years

2. **How does her history of breastfeeding for three years affect her risk for osteoporosis?** It doesn't. Although women will deplete some calcium during the time they are breastfeeding, this is quickly corrected after they wean the babies.

3. **How does breastfeeding affect her risk for breast cancer today?** Breastfeeding reduces the risk for breast cancer in premenopausal woman, but it does not affect her risks today.

4. Define menometrorrhagia. Excessive or irregular menstrual bleeding.

5. Does Josephine need a PAP smear today? No. It is not recommended for women who have had hysterectomies unless they are identified as being at high risk for vaginal cancer, such as having a history of reproductive cancer or having been DES exposed.

6. What other screening test are appropriate for her at this visit? Other tests she should have done include bone density, cholesterol levels, CBC, thyroid function, glucose screen, screening for colon cancer, and mammogram.

7. How does surgical menopause differ from natural menopause? Because surgical menopause is abrupt, the symptoms can be more severe and last longer. Since a woman who has experienced surgical menopause has reduced estrogen levels for a longer period of time, she is also at a higher risk for osteoporosis and heart disease.

8. What effect does her five years on HRT have on her health risk for heart disease? For the first years she was on HRT she was at a higher risk for a heart attack. Evidence today does not support the use of HRT for prevention of heart disease.

9. What effect does her five years on HRT have on her health risk for osteoporosis? During the time she was on the HRT she would have been at a reduced risk for bone loss. However, once she discontinued it she lost any benefits. Therefore, today she is at the same risk as if she had never been on it.

10. What resources can you suggest to help with her financial and living situation? There may be a church group (Catholic charities), United Way organization, Meals on Wheels, or a local group nearby that can help her and still assure her independence.

11. Develop a teaching plan to help Josephine minimize her health risk.
- *Nutrition*
  Review what she eats
  Review how much she can spend on food
  Help her to identify those foods that are highest in nutrients and lowest in cost (high calcium)
  Can she afford calcium supplements?
  Teach her to avoid sodas, especially colas and root beers; caffeine; alcohol; excessive animal proteins; sodium; and refined sugars
  Include foods high in fiber in her daily intake
  Review food preparation with her (avoid reheating foods as they will lose their nutritive value)
  Avoid high fat foods

- *Safety*
  It sounds like she is developing vertebral osteoporosis
  Review posture. Discuss back braces or supports and resources for obtaining needed equipment
  Review the need for night lights, reducing accidents
  Check to see if she needs glasses to see better
  Install railings in her bathtub

How is her memory? Does she remember when she puts food on to cook, turns the iron on, etc?

Does she drive? How is her driving?

Teach her to do a breast self-exam and the warning signs of cancer

■ *Exercise*

What type of exercise does she like?

Where can she exercise?

Are there exercises she can do at home?

Is there someone who can exercise with her?

Determine how much and for how long she should exercise (cardiovascular, muscular, and skeletal assessments)

Include weight-bearing exercise to help her build bone and reduce bone loss

■ *Communication*

Encourage more open communication with her children, who may be willing and able to help her.

References

Morgan, G., & Hamilton, C. (2003). *Practice guidelines for obstetrics and gynecology* (2nd ed.). Philadelphia: Lippincott, Williams & Wilkins.

Whitney, N., Cataldo, C. B., & Rolfer, S. R. (2002). *Understanding normal and clinical nutrition.* Belmont, CA: Thomson/Wadsworth Learning.

Index

Page numbers in **bold** indicate figures.

249